NEW TRENDS IN HEALTH SCIENCES EDUCATION, RESEARCH, AND SERVICES

The McMaster Experience

Edited by
J. F. Mustard; V. R. Neufeld;
W. J. Walsh; J. Cochran

PRAEGER

PRAEGER SPECIAL STUDIES • PRAEGER SCIENTIFIC

Library of Congress Cataloging in Publication Data

Main entry under title:

New trends in health sciences education,
  research, and services.

  Bibliography: p.
  Includes index.
  1. Medical education—Ontario.
2. Paramedical education—Ontario.
3. Medical research—Ontario.   4. Medical
care—Ontario.   5. McMaster University.
Faculty of Health Sciences.   I. Mustard, J. F.
R749.A6N48   610'.7'1171352   82-558
ISBN 0-03-061966-1   AACR2

Published in 1982 by Praeger Publishers
CBS Educational and Professional Publishing
a Division of CBS, Inc.
521 Fifth Avenue, New York, New York 10175 U.S.A.

23456789 052 987654321

Printed in the United States of America

CONTENTS

THE ISSUES: AN OVERVIEW

INTRODUCTION

by J. FRASER MUSTARD, M.D.
Vice-President (Health Sciences)
McMaster University
Hamilton, Ontario, Canada

Since the School of Medicine program was launched at McMaster in
1965, we have had a series of interactions, both here and elsewhere with
faculty from other institutions, particularly the new medical schools.
Many of my colleagues felt that it might be useful if, at some time in
the future, we could bring together faculty from the different schools to
discuss some of the common issues we all face. Also, there have been
various networks of new schools developed within continents and across
continents and in some cases involving all continents. At meetings of
these various groups the suggestion was made from time to time that,
since we are one of the oldest "new schools", we might like to host a
meeting to outline what we have done and to discuss common issues and
problems. Through the efforts of Dr. William Walsh and his colleagues we
have been able to bring you together for this meeting. We have used, as
one reason for holding the meeting at this time, the fact that the
1979-80 academic year marks the tenth year of our admission of the first
class of medical students for the academic year 1969-1970.

It might be helpful for those of you who are not familiar with
McMaster University and Hamilton to provide a brief history. McMaster
University came to Hamilton fifty years ago from the University of
Toronto and will be celebrating its 50th anniversary of the move in the
1980/81 academic year. The University is old by Canadian standards; it
was started in the last century as an affiliated university in the
University of Toronto. However, it has a young history in health
sciences. In 1946, it established a School of Nursing with Gladys Sharpe
as its first director. She subsequently became director of nursing at
Toronto Western Hospital, but before she left she laid a firm foundation

1

for nursing and future developments in health sciences. The School of
Medicine came into being in 1965, when John Evans arrived as its first
dean and started to bring together a group of people to create a School
of Medicine, with the idea that it would become part of a Faculty of
Health Sciences involving both Nursing and Medicine. We are, as you
know, a Faculty of Health Sciences which has a number of education
programs, two of which are Undergraduate Nursing and Undergraduate
Medicine. When we established the School of Medicine we recognized that
we had an opportunity to establish new approaches to academic medicine
within a university which had a tradition of doing things a bit
differently. It is important to indicate that the university climate at
that time under President Thode was not negative to what we wanted to do;
it was, in fact, quite positive.

In establishing the program in Undergraduate Medicine we reviewed
some of the problems all of us had faced within our former institutions
and some of the problems that had been brought to the attention of those
of us in academic medicine from a number of jurisdictions. At that time,
some medical educationalists, economists, sociologists and others were
very strong in their criticisms of medicine. Among the problems
identifed were the following:

1.   Rigid, lock-step curricula in which the amount of time for
various subjects, the nature of the curriculum and the methods for
presenting material to students was determined by a) the power of
departments, b) the past history of departments in the control of
curricula, and c) the administrative structure of the school. Those who
had been there the longest with the tightest control of the dean's office
often had the best control of the curriculum.

2.   A sharp distinction between pre-clinical and clinical medical
sciences which inhibited the use in the pre-clinical part of medical
education of staff in clinical departments who had a good understanding
of human physiology.

3. An imbalance in the exposure of students to health problems as seen within an active treatment hospital in terms of acute health problems, and to health problems as seen among the general population in the community. In the 1960's the general practitioner was generally considered, in many jurisdictions, to be a disappearing physician in the provision of health care.

4. A divergence in the goals of the university faculties of medicine and the teaching hospitals and their staff. Often the goals attributed to the faculty were really the goals of isolated departments who used the name of the university with the hospital administration to achieve their objectives in the teaching hospital. There often was no coordinated approach between the schools of medicine and the administrative structure in the teaching hospitals in terms of planning and the recruitment of staff, which led to varying degrees of ill-feeling, misunderstanding and distortions in the use of resources, duplication of facilities, etc.

5. The view that medical research was largely irrelevant. Faculty were not concerned with assessing the effectiveness of diagnostic and treatment procedures, and no one was studying the efficiency with which effective health care was delivered.

6. A lack of concern in the education programs with the preparation of physicians to provide sensitive, effective, efficient primary care in the community.

This is a partial list of the criticisms that were common in the 1960's. Some of these are ones with which all of you are familiar. Some of them may be new, and some may be peculiar to our Ontario setting.

When we began trying to set up arrangements so that the Medical School could address some of these issues, we were uncertain what to do. Although we did not have any profound insight, we had two advantages. We were small and therefore could easily discuss the problems and potential solutions wich each other, and we had a very sympathetic University led by its president, Dr. Harry Thode. We stumbled into a number of arrangements through trial and error that allowed us to undertake some new approaches.

We developed an administrative arrangement whereby the education programs would be the responsibility of the Faculty, particularly in relation to policies and review of the programs. This prevented the education programs from being controlled by departments.

We established our research programs as a Faculty initiative as far as policy priorities and resource management are concerned.

We worked with the hospitals and other institutions in Hamilton which provided health care to set up arrangements to allow conjoint planning and open discussion of problems, no matter how difficult. We found ways to come to a reasonable solution to most problems, taking into account the fact that each of the teaching hospitals and health care units (such as the Public Health Unit in which nurses would be educated) are autonomous units. We created our own form of health council for district planning of health services long before the Government created district health councils.

An early outcome of these arrangements was the establishment of broadly-based education programs in all sectors of health care, both locally and in remote parts of the province. Within these arrangements it was expected that a student should be able to achieve a balanced view of the different sectors of health care, and also achieve some idea of the issues that relate to population health as a whole as opposed to individual health. The student, by the time he or she finished the undergraduate program, should be in a position to identify the primary issues in a health problem and secure and apply the relevant knowledge to solve the problem, taking into account the roles of different professionals in the health and social sciences. The student was expected to have a good understanding of the scientific basis of medicine and be able to assess critically the evidence concerning the causes of ill-health and the merits of the various diagnostic and treatment procedures.

The education program that was established provides for considerable flexibility, but places considerable demand on the student for his or her own education. We called it "problem-based learning" or "self-directed learning," and while it may be a bit new for medicine, this approach has been used for the humanities in institutions such as Oxford and Cambridge for a long time. A key problem that has emerged out of this educational approach is, of course, the question of how to evaluate students in comparison to students in more traditional programs.

A second outcome was the development of arrangements in research which cut across traditional departments and allowed for some integration of basic, applied, and health care research. For example, we have a professor of biochemistry who is interested in what happens to cells when they are exposed to chemicals, which of course is toxicology, and the relationship of this to cancer. He is now applying some of the results of the basic work to the identification of mutagens in the air around the coke ovens in our steel plants and the presence of mutagens in the urine of steelworkers. As you might expect, the air samples from the work areas where there is a high risk of cancer contain high levels of mutagens. We have other areas where our research groups embrace a spectrum of activities from basic to applied research. This research approach requires the faculty to support selected areas of research with an appropriate concentration of resources, and necessitates the establishment of suitable arrangements with the various institutions to do applied research.

To achieve all of these goals it was clear that we needed an effective partnership arrangement between ourselves and all the teaching hospitals. This is complex, because each hospital is independent and has its own Board of Governors or Trustees. The primary institutions are the Hamilton Civic Hospitals (Hamilton General and Henderson General), St. Joseph's Hospital, and the Chedoke-McMaster Hospital (the Chedoke Division, and the McMaster Division which occupies 60 percent of the Health Sciences Centre). How does one work out satisfactory partnership

relationships which take into account the responsibilities of the
institutions for providing care and the responsibility of the university
in providing its academic programs? In Canada it is generally agreed
that clinical staff should hold joint appointments in the hospital and in
the university. In general, senior academic faculty are chiefs of
service in the teaching hospitals. The question of how to make these
appointments and periodically review them is complicated. We had an
advantage in that we were new and had good cooperation with our community
and its institutions. We do have a large faculty and this is the result,
in part, of the fact that the community and its institutions have worked
with the Faculty of Health Sciences to establish joint programs in health
care, teaching and research, and of jointly-made arrangements to recruit
the appropriate staff.

A key element in the recruitment and motivation of faculty was the
development of a system of rewards related to the objectives of our
programs. We could not be tied to narrow university requirements for
promotion, tenure and salary increases based on research alone. We felt
education was important and that it would have to be recognized. We also
recognized that contributions to health service by faculty in clinical
departments was important and that these activities should be monitored,
assessed and be part of faculty evaluation. We managed to get our
University to accept the premise that a faculty member could be promoted
to full professor if the faculty member was recognized (nationally) to be
a distinguished senior physician in his or her specialty area. Our
Faculty operations require considerable effort on the part of faculty to
make things work. This "administration" – not administration in the
sense of a dean or a department chairman, but administration in terms of
making programs work – is also recognized in promotion, tenure and salary
settlements. Thus a faculty member can be rewarded because of his work
in research, education, or health services, taking into account
contributions to the operation of Faculty programs. Normally a faculty
member is expected to contribute in education and in either research or
health services.

6

Finally, the Health Sciences Centre was designed with consideration of all these various points. We did not want the students to be isolated in pre-clinical and clinical sectors of the building, nor did we want Nursing and Medicine to be isolated. We wanted to have an environment in which the learning resources would be readily available for students at all levels of education. The result has been a building which houses a hospital with a large ambulatory care service, and everything else that goes with an academic health sciences faculty and a clinical teaching centre. The building is owned by the University, and the hospital portion is leased to Chedoke-McMaster Hospital, which operates the hospital.

For this meeting we have chosen four major themes for discussion:

1. Networks. What kind of health service or health sciences networks should schools of medicine and faculties of health sciences be in their community? Should they be integrated as best they can with the institutions in their community to provide a broad spectrum of health care from community to institutional base for clinical education, or should health science centres be separate empires, isolated from the rest of the system?

2. Education. How should education be handled within such a framework? Where should the responsibilities reside for the education programs? Who should have the responsibility for undergraduate education? Who should have the responsibility for the training of graduates in specialized areas of medicine? We use the term "postgraduate medicine" in our jurisdiction. The university has the responsibility in Canada, but in other jurisdictions you will find other groups with the responsibility.

3. Research. How strong should the research base be, and what relationship should there be with the system as a whole in terms of basic research, applied research (testing of whether new knowledge is valuable) and research directed towards determining whether useful knowledge can be

more efficiently provided in the provision of health care (which in the health care field is a very key issue)?

4. <u>Motivation and Preparation</u>. A key to making everything work in a faculty of health sciences is reasonable motivation and preparation of the people who are involved in the programs. "Faculty motivation" is a rather narrow term, because there is more than faculty involved in a system such as this; there are the staff in the hospitals and the other institutions who are important. One has to understand the importance of their participation and recognition in the health sciences programs.

I have given you a brief historical background of this institution and its academic programs and an explanation of why we have chosen to examine the four themes at this meeting. In terms of our experience, it is these themes that have been important in our ability to establish flexible arrangements which maximize the opportunities to develop strong programs in the health sciences.

THE ISSUES: AN OVERVIEW

THE HEALTH SCIENCES NETWORK

by A. QUERIDO, M.D.
Professor, Akademisch Ziekenhuis Leiden
The Netherlands

I would like to offer my sincere congratulations to your Faculty of
Health Sciences on the tenth anniversary of the admission of the first
class in Medicine at McMaster University. It must be most stimulating
for a faculty to be aware that its endeavour for new teaching methods in
medical education and its efforts to fit this education into an existing
health care system have attracted the world-wide attention of medical
educators. This is a very significant feat! I am most honoured to be
invited as a guest speaker.

The "health sciences network," taken literally, is concerned with
education and research; otherwise it would not be a "science" network.
However, it is so intertwined with the health care network that it is
impossible to talk about the first without considering the last. There
are many reasons for the interdependence of health sciences and medical
care, of which I will discuss only two. In the first place, prevention
and health services, especially the latter, are predominantly an activity
of humans. It is therefore not astonishing that 80 percent of the total
cost in the health care system goes toward salaries. Individual
performance is a major factor in the quality of the health care network.
In the second place, whatever one thinks of universities, there is a
concentration of knowledge and skills there which should also be
available for public service and which can be, through its quality, a
driving innovative force.

If my discussion were limited to speaking about Ontario, many things
would not have to be said because they are discussed in the impressive
monograph series of the Ontario Council of Health.[1] I was asked,
however, to approach the problem in a more general way.

9

The Health Care System

For many reasons, there is no such thing as an "ideal" health care system. Such systems have developed everywhere in different ways, and each bears the marks of its past. A kind of general theory of health care, however, has recently emerged. The impetus was provided in Western industrialized countries by the unmanageable costs, and in the developing countries by the absence of a health care system and the extremely limited funds available for its development. In considering this theory, however, one should be aware that any theory about a service system is based upon comparisons, analogies, a few facts, and much wishful thinking.

The health care system of Western countries is so large that it consumes 8-10 percent of the gross national product and employs 5-6 percent of the labour force. Three subsystems can usually be identified: that which deals with environmental health problems; that which deals with self care and primary care, as it is called by the World Health Organization (WHO); and that which lodges sick people for diagnosis, treatment and care, which for simplicity I will call the "hospital-based" system.

Environmental health services aim mainly at preserving or creating a harmless environment: clean water, clean soil and air, and adequate clean food. They concern themselves with groups of people and those factors which impinge on health but which must be managed collectively. In the past, "environmental health" has been equated, if not confounded, with "public health," and it has also been concerned with problems of communicable diseases, mental health and social services. Sometimes special categories of programs have been included, such as those directed against alcoholism or tuberculosis. Since environmental health is concerned with groups and with the population in general, its funding is mainly through central, provincial or local governments. It is the subsystem that, together with economic development, has contributed most to the increase of life expectancy.

10

Primary care usually means self-care or care by aides and
auxiliaries in the developing world, and it means continuous contact
between health professionals and a relatively small subset of the
population in the developed world. It deals with most of the problems of
the individuals seeking care at that level. It is intertwined with the
psychosocial and social medical services. Because its structure is
rooted in the cultural and political development of the country, it is
the least comparable of the three subsystems from one country to
another. Countries like Great Britain and Holland are well supplied with
primary care units or multi-units, with one doctor for every two thousand
to three thousand inhabitants. In such countries, the primary care
system functions as an entrance to the entire health care system. In
developing countries, primary care is recommended (WHO Alma-Ata meeting[2]
and Organization for Economic Cooperation and Development) as the first
priority in the development of the health care systems. In
industrialized countries the major concern is the medicalization of
social problems. Although in many settings primary care workers have
access to beds in health centres and hospitals, the service is basically
ambulatory and community based.

The hospital-based network with small and large hospitals is the
most costly part of the system, and in Western countries generally
absorbs two-thirds of the equipment and resources of the entire system.
Hospitals should be defined functionally according to the number of
specialties each has and the size of its catchment area. The size of the
specialty services determines their technical and medicotechnical infrastructure, and is an important factor in the day-to-day cost of the
particular hospital.

These three subsystems should be integrated into a flexible total
care system. As I said earlier, the development of the entire system and
its costs have been tumultuous because of increases in the variety of
technical and scientific interventions possible and the vast economic
investments and increasing demands which are generated by them. Since

11

80 percent of the cost goes toward salaries for personnel, manpower
planning is one of the major instruments for giving form to the structure
of the health care system and for cost containment. The goal for the
total system should be the availability to the entire population of
whatever can be offered economically by the country. Whatever is done in
the health care system, therefore, should be both efficient and
efficacious, in order to provide the widest possible range of beneficial
services for the entire population served.

It is well known that the quality of medical care in a country
cannot be adequately measured by the ratio of doctors to inhabitants.
There are countries with one doctor for each four thousand inhabitants
where we would prefer not to be treated. It is instead the number and
ratio of personnel in all branches - doctors, midwives, nurses, physio-
therapists, technicians, etc . - that determine the quality of the
medical care system. I do not intend to make comparisons of the numbers
employed in the different health professions between countries with
different backgrounds and incomes. I would instead find it instructive
to discuss the extreme example of a developing country, because it
illustrates the problems of manpower planning so dramatically.

I have suggested that the amount of money available in goods and
services for health services depends upon the wealth of the country.
This axiom applies to both of the largest service systems: the education
system and the health care system. Where the national per capita income
of a country is $200 per year, the country will spend no more than
1 percent, i.e. $2 per person, for health. On the other hand, a wealthy
country (like Holland, my own country) with a per capita income of $9,000
per year spends 8-10 percent, i.e. $800 per person, on health care. If
the health care system is not nationalized, this money comes not from the
national budget but mainly through insurance arrangements.

The challenging question is how the developing country can best
spend its $2 per person to optimize the benefits. If the decision is
made that $1 should go to environmental health services (the most

effective approach), 50 cents to hospitals, and 50 cents to primary care, it is still possible to achieve a great deal. Assume that there is one doctor available per 50,000 people and that this academically-trained person is put in charge of a health centre for those 50,000 people. At the rate of 50 cents per person for primary care, there will be $25,000 available for this activity. The long educational period of the doctor (about 17 years!) and his expectations entitle him to, say, a salary of $7,500 per year. If the costs of the supplies for the centre are $5,000, that still leaves $12,500 for other health professionals. If the required period of education for several other functions is shortened, it would become possible to pay eight or ten other people. There might, for instance, be two nurses or medical assistants with training periods of nine or ten years (i.e. basic education, some secondary education, and three years of professional training). There would also be room for two midwives whose duties would include supervising "untrained" midwives of the villages. There would also be enough money for a specialist in sanitation, a laboratory technician with a total of eight years' education, an administrator, a pharmaceutical assistant, a driver, and others. The leaders in the villages (teachers, religious leaders), who act as volunteers, would be instructed by the health centre about ways to transfer information and practices based on health education and family planning to the population. In an area where the life expectancy is about forty years and the "under-five" mortality is 30 percent, such a system could effectively change these figures to a life expectancy of fifty years and an "under-five" mortality of a few percent. It should be stressed, however, that the role and function of the doctor in charge of the health centre, which is in large part managerial, is in my opinion more difficult than that of a heart surgeon in a well-staffed hospital with an adequate infrastructure!

TABLE 1

```
┌─────────────────────────────────────────────┐
│              PRIMARY CARE PERSONNEL           │
│              (Industrialized Countries)       │
│                                               │
│              1 doctor per 2,000 people        │
│                                               │
│   $150 per capita available                   │
│      for services and drugs:                  │
│                                               │
│                     1 doctor                  │
│                     1 district nurse          │
│      Services:      midwife                   │
│                     physiotherapist           │
│                     dietitian                 │
│                     psychosocial personnel    │
│                     medico-social personnel   │
│                                               │
│                                               │
│      ─────────────────────────────────        │
│                                               │
│   plus backup environmental health services   │
└─────────────────────────────────────────────┘
```

TABLE II

```
┌─────────────────────────────────────────────┐
│          PRIMARY CARE PERSONNEL               │
│          (Developing Countries)               │
│                                               │
│        1 doctor per 50,00 people              │
│                                               │
│  50 cents per capita available = $25,000      │
│                                               │
│     1 doctor                    $ 7,500       │
│                                               │
│     2 nurses                                  │
│     2 midwives                                │
│     1 sanitation technician                   │
│     1 laboratory technician     $12,500       │
│     1 pharmacy assistant                      │
│     1 administrator                           │
│     1 driver                                  │
│                                               │
│     Materials                   $ 5,000       │
│                                               │
│     ───────────────────────────────          │
│                                               │
│     plus village workers                      │
└─────────────────────────────────────────────┘
```

I think that this extreme example shows clearly what we are up
against in our systems. In my country there are only dispensing
opticians; qualified optometrists do not exist. The optometrical tasks
are assumed by the ophthalmologist, of whom there is 1 per 40,000
people. In Great Britain, where there are well-trained ophthalmic
opticians, there is 1 ophthalmologist for every 100,000 people. The
Dutch ophthalmologists claim to be overworked, and insist upon increasing
their numbers! On the other hand, in Holland 40 percent of all
deliveries are still performed by well-trained midwives, and the only
country which has a lower perinatal death rate is Sweden! These examples
show that manpower planning for the health care system cannot be done by
the profession alone; it must also be a responsibility of local,
intermediate and central governments. The obstacles, of which historical
background, expectations of the population, and the personal interests of

the health professions are only some, are great. But without manpower planning on a national basis and consideration of the ensuing demands on the educational system, it is impossible to achieve the best, most efficient and efficacious health care system available within the means of a country.

The first recommendation of an Organization for Economic Cooperation and Development (OECD)-Expert Committee in 1975[3], accepted by the OECD Council, stated that:

> Clearly expressed national health policies should be developed, preferably by permanently-established planning mechanisms in which providers and consumers of health play a participatory role.

But what are the objectives of a satisfactory health care system and what are the means for achieving them? I will confine my discussion to an indication of only some of the problems. When the system has to answer "needs and demands," how are "needs" defined? This is not difficult for a developing country where the problems are quite clear (life expectancy, perinatal death, crude mortality, etc.), but for a healthy, industrialized country, problems of definition abound. Canada is fortunate to have its Lalonde Report[4] to define health care needs. When we use the term "needs," we apply a normative terminology. Is the objective to prolong life expectancy, to prevent illness, or to improve the quality of life, etc.?

What are the "means" for achieving objectives? Table III shows that in 1978 when the health care system in The Netherlands consumed 26 billion guilders (9% of GNP), the population also consumed 8.6 billion guilders of tobacco, soft drinks and alcoholic beverages. This raises the question of whether a society's legislation for health care should cover everything for everybody, or whether it should leave options open for separate insurance coverages, so that people could choose between whiskey, tobacco, or a bypass operation.

16

TABLE III

SOME DUTCH DATA ON NATIONAL EXPENDITURES
AND LIFE EXPECTANCY

	1953	1978
Health % GNP	3.1	8.6
Education % GNP		6.8
Soft and alcoholic drinks + tobacco % GNP		2.8
Life expectancy years from birth		
— males	70.9	72
— females	73.5	78.4

Although there is an abundance of literature discussing these problems and their macro-economic consequences, the preceding discussion shows clearly that governments have to choose, because otherwise they cannot create intermediate and long-term policies which will:

1) provide in a timely way an educational system which can perform its tasks satisfactorily, and

2) keep open the possibility for new scientific developments in health through cost containment of the existing facilities.

For a country in its totality these problems are overwhelmingly complex. It was the merit of the Dawson Report of 1920[5] and the Goodenough Report in 1944,[6] indicating the importance of education for the health services, and the foresight of Grant in China, Bhore in India and Engel (1958) in Sweden in understanding the central importance of the regionalization of health services that made the analysis of the problems, and the implementation of solutions, operational through practical definitions and applications of regionalization. In 1968 the British Todd Report[7] proposed a structure for the governing relations of the university hospital group within a regional hospital service (which was considered an improvement over what had emerged in the years after 1950). In 1969 the Ontario Council of Health[8] in a report on regional organization of health services recommended:

> . . . that such a regional health organization should be based, in general and where specifically applicable, on university spheres of influence and interest and that every reasonable means be taken to assure that the health sciences centres of these universities are capable of assuming an active dual role in education and research, as is their prime function, as well as in continuing education, re-training and service consulting in both the professional and semi-professional aspects of the total health services with which they may be totally or in part responsible.

And finally the previously mentioned OECD-Expert Committee of 1975, whose conclusions were approved in 1976 by the OECD Council, put forward in recommendations 2 and 3:

> 2. National health care policies should foster conjoint education/ health care action at the regional level, and institutions at that level should establish mechanisms to implement such actions.
>
> 3. Permanent means of co-ordinating and integrating government action in health care and education of the health professions should be established.

Although the number of member countries in the OECD (all industrialized nations) which have acted upon these recommendations is very limited, the scene seems to be definitely set. It should be stressed that the foregoing definitions of a region are based upon a "complete set" of health care facilities together with all related teaching facilities, including a university. How many of these "complete sets" there are in a country again depends upon the national income. In Western industrialized countries, the size of a region is about 1-2 million people.

The Health Sciences Network

The basic setting for productive cooperation between the health care system and the educational system (i.e. the "health sciences network") and the basis for manpower planning, improvement of quality, and cost containment, can be defined theoretically. That does not, however, mean that all the problems have been solved.

Intense cooperation is required between these two large systems, and Dr. Fraser Mustard has taught me this can only happen if three main conditions are fulfilled: adequate legislation, accountability, and compliance. Legislation is necessary because it stems from national objectives and provides the framework for governance and for responsibilities in both the administrative and financial spheres. Accountability is necessary to maintain quality control. Compliance is necessary to make everything work, because educational and research efforts cannot be extorted. It is also important to recognize that teaching takes time, and this time commitment cannot always be obtained from volunteer teachers. Teaching requires preparation and contact hours with students, whether individually, in small groups, or in lectures. The time required for clinical teaching is hard to analyze, because it includes an element in addition to teaching from which the patient also profits. Although it is not always possible to make a clear distinction between these different activities, agreement should be reached about the sharing of costs involved. There are many studies and examples showing how to handle this problem of costs.[9,10,11,12] One factor in the financial sphere which is often overlooked is that patient care in teaching hospitals or in other health care facilities such as health centres is more costly than in non-teaching hospitals. This is also a

19

complex problem which has been discussed in the Report of the Royal Commission on the National Health Services in 1979.[13] The report states that the extra cost is only partly due to the teaching activities; it is also the result of higher standards of treatment and care. "The teaching hospital costs contain an element which is impossible to clarify, attributable to excellence." Here also, agreement should be reached between those responsible for teaching and the authorities responsible for health care.

Before discussing objectives for the framework of legislation, some remarks on medical education should be made. The first turning point in medical education was the notion that medical education should not be seen as a preparation for a lucrative private enterprise. The next change, and the most important in my opinion, was the awareness that undergraduate medical education should not be considered a professional training, but rather should be directed toward scientific education, just as in other undergraduate disciplines. The professionalization would follow in the form of postgraduate training, for primary care physicians as well as for specialists. The upsetting fact emerged, however, that postgraduate education (in this case the professionalization phase) was as costly as the undergraduate period! This fact, together with the increased costs for patient care in teaching hospitals and the costs of other teaching facilities, is the big issue in all but a few countries.

Objectives of National Legislation

National legislation, in my opinion, can have only one objective: how to guarantee the best medical undergraduate, postgraduate and continuing education, in order to get the most efficient and efficacious health services for the population. The legislation should indicate who is responsible for what, and who pays in the continuum from undergraduate through postgraduate and continuing education. A combination of existing trends and my own wishful thinking about responsibilities and funding are summarized in Table IV. It does not deal with the nature of that funding, whether through national, insurance, or private funds.

20

TABLE IV

RESPONSIBILITES AND FUNDING SOURCES FOR THE MEDICAL EDUCATION CONTINUUM

Education	Responsibility			Funding	
	University	Profession	Health	University	Health
Undergraduate		+		+	
Postgraduate/ Professionalization	+	+	?		+
Recurrent	+	+	+		+
Other health professionals*	?	+	+	?	+
* depends on structure of education system					

The health services must understand that education, training and continuing education are major factors in an adequate health care system. A medical teaching institution cannot function well unless it is at least an equal partner in the governance of the facilities of institutions it needs for teaching. This holds true for the entire continuum and not just the university hospital. University participation in governance (and therefore also in the choice of manpower and its composition) should apply not only to a university hospital, but also to community hospitals, to local environmental health institutions, and to health centres where education and training occur, even if these constitute only a part of all health facilities for the region. That is the extent of my wishful thinking.

Comparision of the Education and Health Care Delivery System

Finally, a personal remark. The two service systems for education and health have much in common. A number of simplified characteristics are shown in Table V.

TABLE V

```
+------------------------------------------------------------+
|            ROUGH COMMON CHARACTERISTICS IN                 |
|          THE EDUCATIONAL AND HEALTH CARE SYSTEMS           |
|                                                            |
|   - Size determined by level of wealth of country          |
|                                                            |
|   - Operation on principles of "needs" and "demands"       |
|                                                            |
|   - Activities mainly individual efforts                   |
|                                                            |
|   - Eighty percent of budget determined by salaries        |
|                                                            |
|   - Stratified into primary, secondary, tertiary           |
|       educational or health facilities                     |
|                                                            |
|   - Quality control difficult                              |
|                                                            |
+------------------------------------------------------------+
```

Both systems are linked by an extension of the meaning given to "human rights." With some imagination, one can see social and political actions directed against illiteracy (such as compulsory primary education circa 1900) as comparable to the promotion of health (WHO, 1948) and its implementation through primary care for all (WHO Alma-Ata, 1978). If this comparison is accepted, it becomes clear that the minimum duties for governmental action in the health field involve four functions:

1. Environmental health services.
2. Creation of legislative and financial conditions for providing primary care for the entire population.
3. Legislation which guarantees facilities, teaching resources and financing for the entire medical educational continuum.
4. Development of a flexible system for health manpower planning.

22

Looking at the health care system in this way has clarified several problems for me. If such a view can withstand criticism, I hope it will have a similar effect for others. We are familiar with the idea that the educational system is open-ended, and that in different countries different solutions have been proposed to answer the problems created by the open-ended approach. The functions and interventions of governments can be identified as regulatory and/or concerned with creating a framework for flexible development.

Educational activities of an advanced nature are very much interrelated with research activities, whether of the teacher or the trainee. Although these activities are essential elements in the development of the "health sciences network," the complexity of decisions in this field and the difficulty of comparing the structures in which scientific endeavour operates in different countries made me decide to omit this aspect, for the sake of clarity.

Acknowledgement

My sincere thanks go to Kerr L. White, M.D. of the Rockefeller Foundation for his stimulation, reading of the manuscript and many helpful suggestions for improving the text.

References

[1] Report on the Health Planning Task Force (Chairman: J.F. Mustard), Ontario Ministry of Health, 1974.

[2] International Conference on Primary Health Care, Alma-Ata, 1978.

[3] New Directions in Education for Changing Health Care Systems. OECD, Paris, 1975.

[4] Canada, Department of Health and Welfare. A New Perspective on the Health of Canadians. Marc Lalonde. Ottawa, 1974.

[5] Ministry of Health (1920). Consultative Counsel on Medical and Allied Services, Interim Report on the Future Provision of Medical and Allied Services. (Dawson of Penn Report) (London: HMSO).

[6] Report of the Interdepartmental Committee on Medical Schools (1968) (Goodenough Report)(London: HMSO).

[7] Report of the Royal Commission on Medical Education 1965–1968 (Chairman: A.R. Todd). HMSO, London, 1968.

[8] Regional Organization of Health Services. Annex A. Report of the Ontario Council of Health. Ontario Department of Health, 1969.

[9] Undergraduate Medical Education: Elements, Objectives, Costs. Committee on the Financing of Medical Education. Association of American Medical Colleges. Journal of Medical Education. 1974b, 49, 101–128.

[10] Report of a Study: Costs of Education in the Health Professions. (Parts 1, 2 and 3). Institute of Medicine. National Academy of Science, Washington, D.C., 1974.

[11] What Accounts for the Higher Costs of Teaching Hospitals? A.J. Culyer, J.W.J. Wisemand, M.F. Drummond, P.A. West. Social and Economic Administration, 1978, 12, nr. 1. pp. 20–30.

[12] Analyzing and Constructing Cost. Meredith A. Gonyea. 1978, Jossey-Bass Inc. San Francisco, Washington, London.

[13] Report of the Royal Commission on the National Health Service (Chairman: Sir Alec Merrison). HMSO, London, 1979, pp. 273–283.

THE ISSUES: AN OVERVIEW

FACULTY MOTIVATION AND PREPARATION

by DAVID MADDISON, M.D.
Dean, Faculty of Medicine
University of Newcastle
New South Wales, Australia

I must confess to finding it somewhat paradoxical and perverse of my esteemed colleagues at McMaster to invite me, as dean of one of the world's newest medical schools, and one that is certainly still in the process of development, to address you on the topic of "Faculty Motivation and Preparation." While I suspect, perhaps unfairly, that even at McMaster there are major issues in this area which still need to be resolved, certainly we in Newcastle could only regard ourselves as entering, at best, the second lap of this particular marathon. I am thus engaged in the bizarre exercise of bringing you coals from Newcastle, in two bags:

(i) Our collective sense of commitment in this sphere, based on a conviction that it is a matter of absolutely central importance, not only for the development of innovative education programs but, even more critically, for the maintenance of the momentum of such innovation.

(ii) A description of the steps that we have already taken, and of some that we are proposing to take, in order to show to the world at large, but most particularly to our own Faculty and our own University, that all faculty members must be properly motivated, prepared and rewarded to ensure the success of the program, without at the same time prejudicing the career development of individual staff members.

The Recruitment of Faculty

Before we examine techniques and programs for the motivation and preparation of faculty, we must first address the issues of recruitment -- issues which, in my part of the world at least, have become progressively more difficult over the past decade or so. From my recent work with

deans from a number of Asian medical schools, I know that this is a very
general problem, possibly afflicting the developing countries even more
adversely than is the case in Canada, Australia and points west.

I imagine that within this audience there would be no serious
argument advanced against the notion that a Faculty should evolve a
coherent educational philosophy, and then wherever possible ensure that
recruitment is substantially influenced by this philosophy. Although the
fear is sometimes expressed that such a recruitment policy might lead to
a dangerously homogeneous collection of staff members, the magnitude of
individual differences between academics is so great that this is never a
realistic threat.

In the implementation of such a recruitment policy, however, there
are many obstacles:

(a) Academic salaries and associated reward systems may not be
competitive, in certain countries at certain times, when related to the
financial gains that may be derived from independent, private practice
and even, in many instances, when compared with the salaries paid to
hospital specialists. To the best of my knowledge, not many countries
experience the freedom accorded to deans of medical schools in North
America, whereby they can be much more sensitive to so-called marketplace
forces when recruiting to particular positions. In Australia the basic
salary offered to a professor of medicine is the same as that offered to
a professor of French, although the former admittedly is granted what is
called a clinical loading, usually $5,000 per annum - a dollop of cream
which, it should be noted, is not available to professors in the
so-called basic sciences, which is one of the reasons, although not the
only reason, why senior recruitment in these disciplines has become so
difficult in recent years. Admittedly there are pickings to be obtained
from consultant practice for many of the senior academics in a faculty of
medicine, but this can all too easily turn into a double-edged sword, as
many third world countries (and not a few first and second world
countries) know to their cost.

26

(b) Because of the considerations that I have just mentioned, and sometimes for other reasons as well, the medical school is not always able to pick and choose from a wide range of available and appropriate candidates for professorial or sub-professorial positions. In many parts of the world, recruitment decisions are even now being taken in order to fill posts which are deemed to be absolutely essential for the faculty to function at all, but which involve individuals who are even at the time quite explicitly recognized by the university as being less than completely suitable.

(c) The traditions of the parent university may result, explicitly or implicitly, in disproportionate weight being attached to the applicant's record in research and scholarship, with his record in the planning and acceptable delivery of exciting education programs being given less attention than it deserves. Faculties of medicine across the world differ quite substantially in the extent to which they are required to conform to the practices of the parent university; in Australia, where the British and in particular the Scottish tradition has never really wavered, it is virtually impossible to award a high-ranking title which somewhere includes the word "professor" unless the individual measures up to the standards that were applied in Edinburgh in 1880. I am not saying that this is necessarily a bad thing, by the way; I simply record that, in this particular dimension, North American medical schools tend to have many more degrees of freedom than their counterparts in other areas of the world. The practical consequence is that in Newcastle, as in all Australian universities and in many other institutions in the Commonwealth, an individual who is of appropriately senior status within his discipline and who is strongly committed to our particular philosophy of education cannot be appointed (or promoted) to senior academic rank if he lacks a significant record of research and scholarship, backed up by a substantial list of publications in international, refereed journals. Even though in this instance the money might be quite irrelevant, a man with thirty years experience in his discipline, nationally and

27

internationally, is not going to feel particularly excited when he kneels before the dean to be dubbed with the title of "clinical lecturer". Please note that I am in no sense implying that research and scholarship are unimportant characteristics of medical academics. Certainly common sense dictates that a medical school will recruit a significant proportion of younger academics whose main claim to attention is a strong research background, and who lack any major involvement in, or commitment to, education up to that time; there is nothing wrong with this, provided that such persons clearly demonstrate a serious commitment to the education program, and to the rapid development of their own skills as educators.

The Retention of Faculty

It is surely self-evident that, in a medical school committed to high quality education, there will be few if any staff members on establishment who can allocate a lavish amount of their time to personal research activities. This may have several important consequences.

(a) Job satisfaction may decline, for academics of high quality inevitably gain a significant quantum of their personal rewards from participation in investigative activity.

(b) The education program may become almost totally identified with vocational training, if it lacks the constant infusion of the new ideas that come from personal participation in the advancement of knowledge.

(c) Academics, particularly those of non-professorial status, may begin to worry, with considerable justification, about the long-term effect of their educational commitment on their own career development. This worry concerns not only their promotion prospects on their own campus, but also their acceptability to another, more traditional, institution if and when they seek a position elsewhere.

It follows therefore that the medical school, and indeed the parent university, must pay proper attention to the development of an appropriate reward system for those who are prepared to commit a substantial proportion of their time to the planning and delivery of an exciting educational program. No one to my knowledge has yet devised a completely satisfactory answer to this problem, for several reasons:

(a) Research publications are not only easily quantified, for what that is worth, but, if published in refereed journals, have by definition been subjected to the impartial judgment of other scholars.

(b) Whatever members of the Faculty of Medicine may think, the parent university may have strong views of its own. It may, for example, take insufficient cognizance of the complex teaching/research/service task which has to be undertaken by most medical school academics, and it may therefore be rather patronizing about the medical academic's achievement when considering applications for promotion.

(c) The nature and extent of the clinician's educational commitments in hospital and community, in particular, are only partially comprehended, at best, in most universities.

(d) There is nothing like universal agreement, and often not much agreement between two universities in the same city, about what characterizes an effective educator; even if such agreement existed, we lack generally agreed scales, known to be both valid and reliable, for the measurement of these characteristics.

Reward for Educational Commitment

I am prepared to go on record, here or anywhere else, that the evaluation of an individual staff member's performance as an educator is one of the toughest assignments, if not the toughest of all assignments, that is brought before the senior staff of an educationally progressive medical school. Of course one can simply be quantitative about it, and such an approach is not altogether to be despised; certainly any dean, and any promotions committee, needs to have available an objective record of the extent to which each individual has participated in the education program, even though he may not always have a crystal-clear perception of what it all means. The more innovative the program, the greater the

29

difficulty: in our own program, with a high commitment to the provision of self-directed, self-monitored learning experiences for the students, the preparation of educational materials is obviously a task of central importance, but much harder to weigh, in an objective way, than a simple head-count of the number of lectures given, seminars conducted and assignments marked.

But we deceive ourselves, and dangerously so, if we do not admit that we are really aiming at some sort of qualitative judgment about each staff member's effectiveness as an educator. There is an enormous literature on this, most of which would be well known to at least the majority of you, and I will not even try to summarize it here. Student evaluation of their teachers, peer review of an individual's educational activities, reports from departmental chairmen, self-evaluation, evaluation of an individual's wirtten materials, prepared either directly for an education assignment or for publication – all have their place, and all have their pitfalls.

In December 1979 I worked in Manila as seminar director for the World Health Organization, planning and implementing the Fourth Regional Seminar on Education and Training for Deans of Medical Schools in the Western Pacific Region. This was an exciting experience, not least because we had as full participants, for the first time, deans from the People's Republic of China, whose experiences and background could hardly be more different from our own. Obviously such a meeting ranged over many of the critical contemporary issues in medical education, but it was stimulating to note how so many deans, from so many different cultures, seized eagerly on the chance to discuss in depth this particular question: the need to develop more refined methods for the evaluation of effectiveness as an educator, leading to how to recognize and reward those staff members who are not only strongly committed to the planning and implementation of the education program, but who are also rated as very effective educators. I can refer only, I fear, to some of the conclusions that we reached, for there is no opportunity here to give you

30

a window on the rich, multicultural discussion that took place. At
least, despite our diverse backgrounds, we could reach agreement that the
performance of teachers must be assessed in the following dimensions:

    (a)   The formulation and communication of clear objectives for the
           segment of instruction.

    (b)   Evidence of thoughtful planning and preparation.

    (c)   Clarity in communication.

    (d)   Enthusiasm for the subject, plus the ability to generate a
           similar enthusiasm in students.

    (e)   Evidence of a thorough understanding of the subject, including
           recent developments therein.

    (f)   Openness to constructive criticism.

Having said all this, however, there was no generally agreed
solution to the "recognition and reward" problem, even when one had
identified a teacher of outstanding commitment and ability. Clearly we
are looking for a commitment from the Faculty, and from the parent
university, to give greatly increased weight to the quality of teaching
(provided that this is accurately assessed) in considering applications
for promotion or for accelerated progression. We discussed at great
length the attention that needs to be given to the composition of
promotion committees, and I was struck by the importance attached in one
country to the inclusion on such committees of non-academic members of
the university's governing body. Some medical schools find that a
"Teacher of the Year" award, determined by student vote, is a valued
technique, but I know of no evidence that it actually motivates staff
members to improve their educational performance. Our Chinese colleagues
laid great emphasis on special awards and citations from high-ranking
officials - but I am inclined to doubt whether, in this country, an
ambitious young academic would gain lasting satisfaction from being
presented by Fraser Mustard with an autographed picture of Pierre
Trudeau. We seem in the West to be rather more preoccupied with

tangible, and in particular financial and status, rewards – but perhaps the Chinese have got it right, and we have got it wrong.

The Preparation of Teachers

Finally, we must briefly consider the self-evident proposition that a university must consider, when it recruits young staff members, not only their training and supervision in the areas of research and scholarship, but also their training and supervision as educators. This is an aspect of medical education which I know has been taken very seriously indeed on this campus, and we would like to think that we are approaching the matter with equal dedication at Newcastle, although I am quite certain that we are a long way yet from getting it right. Certainly we have established a formal Tutor Training Committee, as an offshoot of our Education Committee, and this group, chaired by our professor of medical biochemistry, develops its programs through utilising the skills of a psychiatrist, an internist, a general practitioner and a medical anthropologist. As part of the unwritten "contract" which each tutor, whether full-time or part-time staff, has with the medical school, he or she is required to attend a series of training sessions prior to the first performance as leader of a tutorial group. We have prepared a series of training films for this purpose. It is still too early to conduct a proper evaluation of the extent to which such films, and the discussion that follows them under the leadership of one of our experienced trainers, assist our tutors when they confront such problems in the real life situation, but common sense and anecdotal evidence at this stage suggest that tutors who have been through this program certainly feel better prepared to manage the complex dynamics that inevitably emerge when a collection of bright, somewhat idiosyncratic minds set collectively about the task of problem-solving in groups.

But when one comes to the other end of the journey, and when in our system the dean receives confidential evaluations of the tutors by their students, then a whole new series of problems arise to which we do not even begin to know the answers. What does one do with an influential physician from the community who, despite redoubled efforts to educate him, continues to receive strongly unfavourable reports from his students? One sort of answer is easy, and I assure you that I can, when the time is right, be as ruthless as you would want me to be. On the other hand, I also know, as you know, that the mounting of an innovative education program within a traditional health care system is a highly "political" task, and there is a strict limit to the number of people that one can mortally offend and still maintain the viability of the program.

Conclusion

I suspect that I have said little that is not already known to those of you who have personal experience in the planning, implementation and evaluation of an innovative medical program, within the context of an essentially conservative university system. One of the important factors which operates against the development of sound education programs within a medical school is the existence of a series of outworn stereotypes, prejudices and myths about the teaching and learning process. One has to cope with the disciples of George Bernard Shaw, with his much loved idiot slogan, "He who can does. He who cannot, teaches". This absurd parrot cry encapsulates the worst prejudices of those who wish to give teaching a lowly place in the hierarchy of human tasks, subordinate always to the prestige accorded to the "doer", however irrelevant or even deleterious the deeds might be that he does. One has to fight with the widespread belief that "teachers are born, not made". One has to deal with those many members of our profession who, while they would never dream of claiming that a particular form of therapy was effective in the absence of appropriate supportive evidence, may nevertheless claim to "know", apparently intuitively, all about education.

33

The facts of course are otherwise: unless we are prepared to take education seriously, to recognize that its content and processes are themselves capable of study, research and evaluation, and unless we are prepared to spend as much time, engery and money on the fostering of excellence in education as we do on the fostering of excellence in scholarship and research, then any real prospect of innovative education is beyond us. In my country at least there is an increasing groundswell of dissatisfaction, from the newest student up to our governor general (himself a one-time vice-chancellor), with the low priority accorded to educational excellence in the traditional university. If we can properly harness this criticism and use it for constructive ends, then and only then will we be able to plan, implement and monitor an education program which is truly worthy of those who will be practising doctors in what we hope will be a brave new world.

THE ISSUES: AN OVERVIEW

RESEARCH IN THE HEALTH SCIENCES NETWORK

by Michael Gent, M.Sc.
Asociate Dean (Research), Faculty of Health Sciences
McMaster University
Hamilton, Ontario, Canada

The 10th Anniversary Conference has presented us with an opportunity
to share with each other some of the innovations and frustrations, and
some of the exciting challenges and attempted solutions, which each of us
has had to deal with in recent years in our faculties of health
sciences. It is in this spirit of sharing that I would like to outline
to you some of the objectives and achievements of the Faculty of Health
Sciences at McMaster as they relate to research, and draw attention to
the special nature of the needs, responsibilities and opportunities which
are an inherent part of the health sciences network.

Since there is no uniform definition of "health sciences network,"
let me explain how I have interpreted it. Within the faculty of health
sciences, the network would include 1) the administrative organization
governing the policies and execution of research, 2) the combination of
two or more of the many discipline areas into programmatic activity,
3) the spectrum of research from the development of new knowledge through
the testing of that knowledge to the application of new knowledge, and
4) the interdependence between research, education and service programs.
Beyond the faculty, the health sciences network extends to the rest of
the university, the affiliated hospitals, the local community, the
province, the country, and the rest of the world.

I have not included in this discussion national and provincial
health policies and funding mechanisms, although both are also key
elements.

Administrative Organization

When the founding fathers of our Faculty of Health Sciences at

35

McMaster established a very innovative and exciting MD program, they set out general goals of academic excellence and scholarship which specifically included a strong research base, on the premise that such a base is essential to success in the educational programs and to high quality in health services.

In the present organizational structure of the Faculty, the programs of education, service and research are under the purview of three separate committees, each responsible, through its chairman, to the Dean and Vice-President (Health Sciences) and reporting directly to them and the Faculty Executive and Faculty Council. These committees are advisory rather than executive and thus require approval for any major policy change.

The research committee, called the Committee on Scientific Development (C.S.D.), is chaired by the Associate Dean (Research). The C.S.D. coordinates and facilitates the scientific development of the Faculty of Health Sciences and related programs, gives leadership in the evolution of policy for approval by the Faculty, and discharges an executive function in relation to scientific development. Research is thus organized to a considerable extent along faculty rather departmental lines.

In addition to individual research, the C.S.D. has encouraged the development of research programs of an interdisciplinary and interdepartmental nature. The range of activities of these programs covers basic biological research through to the delivery of health care and the assessment of new procedures.

The C.S.D. also has important administrative functions. Its secretariat sees all research grants before signature by the Associate Dean (Research), advises applicants on budget, resource requirements and possible sources of funding, and arranges ethics review for proposals involving human subjects. It also provides the information base for research for the Faculty.

Several research facilities are centralized under the management of the C.S.D., which in turn is advised by facility managers' and users' committees. These facilities operate on a cost-recovery, fee-for-service basis, and include an analytical ultracentrifuge, animal care facility, biomedical engineering facility, computation services unit, drug analysis laboratory, electron microscopy facility, glasswashing facility, and automatic typewriter service.

The C.S.D. is responsible for the management of resources associated with research, such as space and equipment. It is thus in a position to advise approval or rejection of a grant proposal according to the implications for available resources. In this capacity it attempts to act as a constructive but responsible guardian and facilitator whose objective is to keep the unique university and community health research needs in balance. We believe this centralization of responsibility has resulted in a very efficient use of space and shared facilities.

The C.S.D. also has a responsibility for the display and enforcement of safety regulations -- which is particularly important at this time with the recent introduction of Bill 70 (the Occupational Health and Safety Act, 1978).

Finally, the C.S.D. is responsible for the distribution of certain discretionary funds.

Research Programs

At an early stage, the Faculty identified as one of its prime objectives the development of flourishing research programs which complied with the following three terms of reference:

1. The program should relate to a problem in the area of human biology and health.

2. It should be characterized by as broad a spectrum of interest as possible and should involve multiple departmental and other resources both in its formation and execution.

37

3. The execution of the program should involve synergistic relationships with other programs in education, service and/or research.

In six areas of research, groups have developed to the point where they have received formal recognition by the Faculty as "Research Programs."
These programs are:

1. Cardiovascular Disease, Hemostasis and Thrombosis
2. Host Resistance
3. Reproductive Biology
4. Control of Smooth Muscle Function
5. Brain and Behaviour
6. Educational Development.

In many other research areas there is smaller scale, informal collaboration between various faculty members and their groups. Some of these areas in which the Faculty has strength include respirology; design, measurement and evaluation; occupational health; and toxicology.

The Cardiovascular Disease, Thrombosis and Hemostasis program is, I believe, a good example of the application of the principles of programmatic research. It covers the full range - from the development of new knowledge through its testing by way of clinical trials to its application in practice (e.g. compliance in hypertension and economic aspects of the diagnosis and treatment of deep vein thrombosis). This has resulted in important contributions to developments in diagnosis, treatment and prophylaxis in both venous and arterial thromboembolism.

The Host Resistance program has emphasized immunology research, particularly as it applies to immunological factors in normal pregnancy, the growth and development of the immune system, the special role of immune mechanisms at mucosal surfaces, host-virus interactions, genetics of host defense mechanisms, and host resistance to cancer.

The Reproductive Biology program includes scientists with primary training in biochemistry, endocrinology, anatomy, animal physiology and

38

the veterinary sciences who work in collaboration with clinicians with extended training in biochemistry and physiology. This program has made significant contributions to the understanding of the basic mechanisms of reproduction and has led to changes in the management of labour and the newborn, in the control and enhancement of fertility, and in the management of post-menopausal women.

The Control of Smooth Muscle Function program has as its objective the study of the structural and functional basis for the control of smooth muscle in health and disease. Current activities include studies in control of gastrointestinal and smooth muscle, cardiovascular smooth muscle, myometrium and oviduct, and airway smooth muscle.

The newest program is Brain and Behaviour, in which several groups, primarily from the departments of Neurosciences and Psychiatry, are currently working together in neurobiology, neurotransmission and neuromodulation, and neuropharmacology. Brain and Behaviour is considered to be one of the most exciting areas of research in terms of its potential for a major breakthrough.

Another program which is worthy of particular mention is the Program for Educational Development. This group has made special efforts to apply sound and rigorous methodology in a notoriously "soft" area, and in a financial environment in which few agencies allocate money for such research. A Program Evaluation Group, for example, carries out specific projects related to our own educational programs, including such important studies as the follow-up of McMaster graduates, the performance of McMaster graduates in practice relative to program goals, and the admission process in the MD program. An Evaluation Measures Group carries out specific studies of methods and instruments for the assessment of student performance. A Problem-Based Learning Systems Group carries out projects related to the design, development and evaluation of effective tools for problem-based approaches to learning. And finally, an Educational Studies Group carries out studies involving faculty development and continuing professional education.

Faculty research also has a continuing association and dependence upon many other components in the Health Sciences Network.

The University Component

The Faculty is, of course, an integral part of the University, and as such is expected to contribute to University programs and to take advantage of the opportunity to collaborate with appropriate colleagues from other faculties. A number of inter-faculty funded research projects involve Health Sciences, such as studies of benefit of exercise in post-myocardial infarction patients (with the School of Physical Education), air pollution (with the Department of Engineering), and toxicology (with the Department of Chemistry).

The Hospital Component

The affiliated hospitals play a key role in our research programs, and a high level of collaboration between the hospitals and the University is essential for the establishment of a balanced research environment. The trend to consolidation of health services in particular institutions with a region increases the opportunity to build strong research bases around such services. Research strengths have been established in cardiovascular surgery at Hamiton General Hospital, in respirology and renal disease at St. Joseph's Hospital, and in rehabilitation at the Chedoke Division of Chedoke-McMaster Hospital.

This kind of cooperation produces benefits to all parties involved, and we have good working relationships with the hospitals. The chairmen of the hospital research committees, for example, serve on the C.S.D. There is reciprocity for ethics approval to avoid duplication of effort in multi-hospital studies, and a joint Research Advisory Group serves as the research proposal review committee for both the Faculty of Health Sciences and Chedoke-McMaster Hospital.

About 60 percent of our funded research is basic and 40 percent is clinical and applied. Approximately 70 percent of our research faculty

have their primary base in the Health Sciences Centre – which includes
the McMaster Division of Chedoke-McMaster Hospital – and about 30 percent
are based in other hospitals.

The Community Component

The general community is also a necessary part of the research base,
and several important studies have been carried out in this community
with the help of local physicians. One of these, the "Burlington
Controlled Trial of the Nurse Practitioner," is considered to be a major
technical achievement in health care research. Other studies include
battered children, well-baby care, pre-school assessments, chronic home
care, and air pollution and occupational health.

These studies provide at least indirect benefit to the local
community, but there are direct benefits as well. The Regional Service
Program, which is jointly sponsored by the Health Resources Development
Plan of the Ontario Department of Health and McMaster University,
provides assistance to doctors, nurses, other health professionals, and
health planners and administrators in the McMaster health region who must
make decisions about patient care and health care delivery.

The Regional Service Program gives assistance in the planning,
execution, analysis and interpretation of surveys and other studies
relevant to human biology and health care delivery within the region.
Specifically, it provides trained and experienced personnel in the fields
of clinical epidemiology, health care research methods, health planning,
and medical statistics. These consultations are generally short-term and
may consist of assistance in design of a data-gathering form or an
evaluation. No charge is made for consultation. Since its inception in
1969, the Regional Service Program has provided help in about four
hundred projects.

Resources for this program are drawn mainly from the department of
Clinical Epidemiology and Biostatistics. The members of this group come
from a heterogeneous mixture of disciplines. About half are from

41

clinical disciplines (cardiology, internal medicine, pediatrics, family medicine) and half from non-clinical disciplines (statistics, health economics and psychology). The group is held together by a common interest and expertise in research methodology.

A major objective of this department is the provision of expert advice on the design, execution and analysis of experiments and surveys for a wide variety of research projects originating with members of other departments of the Faculty of Health Sciences – and indeed other departments of the University. Such research projects include biomedical laboratory-based research, clinical therapeutic trials, new conceptual approaches to diagnosis and treatment, and the evaluation of different forms of clinical and community health care. Help has been provided in well over four hundred projects; in many of these, there was simply a provision of service, but for a significant number the project became a collaborative venture between the consultant and the member of the department.

Collaborative Programs

Some of the problems we wish to study cannot be dealt with in our own local community, perhaps because the expertise is not available or not enough patients with certain disorders live in the community. In such circumstances we have sought collaboration with colleagues in other parts of the province. We currently have several joint projects with colleagues from the University of Toronto and other collaborative ventures ongoing with colleagues at the University of Guelph, the University of Waterloo, and the University of Western Ontario in London.

A recent successful collaborative effort on the national level was the Canadian Stroke Study. This was a major six-year study directed by Dr. Henry Barnett from the University of Western Ontario in London, in which investigators from McMaster formed the methods group and coordinating centre. The study, which included twenty-six centres across Canada from Newfoundland to Victoria, showed that aspirin reduced stroke or death among men with transient cerebral ischemia. It also enabled the

42

investigators to learn a great deal clinically from a disciplined and well-documented study of a complex clinical disorder. Other collaborative national studies in cancer and cardiovascular disease are currently in progress.

We have recently established a collaborative program with the University of Laval on health, health care and health policy. The primary objective is to set up a joint capability for consideration of design, measurement and evaluation aimed at the assessment of 1) the effects of environmental and lifestyle factors on human health and the impact of public policy in these areas; 2) the effectiveness and efficiency of health care delivery and appropriate policy; and 3) the impact of financing methods on the scope, quality and efficiency of health care and appropriate policy.

The ultimate use of the network is the establishment of appropriate international research bases, and one need for this is the very large collaborative clinical trial. A particularly important study which is now in progress includes centres in North America, Europe and Japan, and is under the direction of Dr. Henry Barnett from Western and Dr. David Sackett, Dr. Brian Haynes and Mr. Wayne Taylor from McMaster; this study will evaluate the effectiveness of extra-intracranial bypass surgery.

Another equally important reason for international collaboration is the responsibility and opportunity for a school like McMaster to share some of its research resources, particularly the knowledge and skills of established researchers, with less fortunate colleagues in other parts of the world. To this end, we have responded to specific requests from Sierra Leone, South America, Mexico, and the Middle East.

Interaction Between Research and Education

Within the Health Sciences Network, an essential interaction exists between research and education. The objective relating to academic excellence and scholarship in a Faculty of Health Sciences may only be fulfilled when there are real strengths in graduate studies.

43

At this time we have five graduate programs in the Faculty of Health Sciences: Blood and Cardiovascular (MSc, PhD); Growth and Development (MSc, PhD); Neurosciences (MSc, PhD); Design, Measurement and Evaluation (MSc); and Health Care Practice (MHSc). In addition, the department of Biochemistry, which is jointly administered by the Faculties of Science and Health Sciences, has a graduate program, and graduate students in both Science and Health Sciences can take training in biochemistry.

Of these five graduate programs, the first three have specific content areas of specialization in the medical sciences, with fairly conventional objectives for graduate programs. The Design, Measurement and Evaluation program, however, is rather more innovative, with emphasis on methodology appropriate to the full spectrum of health research, while the Master of Health Sciences program is directed towards the enhancement and further development of skills in health care practice.

Attention is currently being directed to the possible conversion of our three existing Medical Sciences programs into a single Faculty program in Medical Sciences, with areas of specialization which match the existing research programs. There is much to be gained by having a common program, such as increased interaction between students in different areas of specialization. Some common needs of students could be met through courses in the architecture of laboratory research and more general courses in human biology and the issues relating to health, health care and health policy.

The Medical Sciences programs have relatively few medical graduates, but the Design, Measurement and Evaluation program has a good mix of clinical and non-clinical people. This particular program has attracted a significant number of residents who take either the whole program or selected courses, as well as several of our Faculty colleagues in the clinical departments.

In recognition of the need to attract medical graduates into research, we encourage our MD students to consider elective experiences in research, and we have recently created an opportunity for a limited number of students to take leave from the MD program to spend time in research.

Conclusions

Universities all over the world are under severe restraints at this time, and the ability to develop and follow up on new opportunities in research is severely limited. This Faculty has established a policy of building on existing strengths in the program areas. We believe it is essential to retain the ability to develop new research capabilities in important areas. Internally, we continue to look for ways in which to provide short-term career support for young investigators; an example of this is the recent establishment of the Rose Levy Rosenstadt Scholar Award by which we hope to be able to support three new research scholars each year for three-year terms. Externally, we are pressing both provincial and federal agencies to devote more money to career support programs. Finally, we would like to develop more space for clinical research, and we are working with our colleagues in the affiliated hospitals to achieve this objective.

The Faculty of Health Sciences at McMaster and the associated health sciences network has been, and is, an exciting environment for health research. We have been fortunate in having stimulating leadership in key areas; in not having to battle with the traditional structures inherent in older medical schools; and in being able to appoint people who recognize the benefits and mutual responsibilities of collaborative research. One of our greatest challenges in the future will be to maintain these opportunities by not allowing barriers to form and indeed by keeping open and strengthening all the links in the health research network.

THE ISSUES: AN OVERVIEW

EDUCATION IN THE HEALTH SCIENCES NETWORK

by Harmen Tiddens, M.D.
Professor, School of Economics, Social Sciences and Law
Tilburg University
The Netherlands

Let me first of all tell you that I feel very honoured and very grateful for this invitation to participate in the 10th Anniversary Conference of the Faculty of Health Sciences of McMaster University. I have great admiration for all that has been achieved here. It was a privilege to meet the founding fathers in the early stages of this enterprise. I reacted in the same way as many people did who were exposed to the enthusiasm and to the vision and logic that characterized this concept: it strongly influenced my thinking about the relationship between medical education and health care and about the relationship that should exist between the objectives for education, research and service within a medical faculty. Many contacts followed, with John Evans and with others in this situation. They were of great help to me in different stages in my career and strongly and visibly influenced my work.

McMaster's Health Sciences Faculty, in close collaboration with those responsible for the health care in the region, created a viable and exciting experiment that, in my opinion, heralded a new era in medical education. Why did it succeed? What were the conditions that favoured its development? I would like to discuss with you some of these conditions as potential issues to be further discussed in the coming days. What prevented other universities, in Europe and in the U.S., from becoming a driving force in the improvement in medical care and health care in the post World War II period? Why did health sciences networks not blossom everywhere?

University Education in the Sixties

At the time when the foundations were laid for this health sciences faculty, universities in the larger part of the industrialized world were wrestling with rapidly growing problems.

TABLE I

THE EXPANSION OF HIGHER EDUCATION IN INDUSTRIALIZED COUNTRIES

	severe entrance selection
population explosion	
	higher standards in examination
expansion – cost explosion –	increased financial contributions
external democratization	shortening of courses
	teacher-independent education
	henk g. schmidt meta media 57, 4-16, 1978

Table I is taken from a publication of Henk G. Schmidt, one of the group of educationalists who played an important role in the development of the Maastricht curriculum. It indicates crucial problems for universities in some industrialized countries, in particular in Europe.

After World War II, in Europe, the barriers that prevented the entry into the university system for the less affluent were rapidly removed. In many countries, legislation did not permit selection procedures for university admission. Everybody with the required qualifications could enter. Universities often grew quite rapidly. University management in general was rather weak; educational expertise was largely lacking. Computer processing of multiple-choice type examinations was about the only educational innovation that was introduced, leading to an increase

47

in the median duration of studies without any indication that there was a benefit in quality.

What were universities facing? An overload of students, weak management, an assignment of a role that they possibly could not and cannot fulfill: the solution to the problem of social inequalities.

Overloaded and underfinanced institutions for higher learning are ill-equipped to bring about change in their own functioning or in the operation of systems like health care.

In addition, student unrest and the political response to it in many countries led to important changes in the structure of universities. Far-reaching democratization often led to a further weakening of university management.

In North America, the basic structure of universities was less forcibly challenged and remained virtually unchanged. There, however, internal conflict between objectives for research, education and service, with a strong predominance of research interests, made educational change difficult to achieve.

In the developing world, the influence of former colonial relationships appeared to be particularly strong in the field of university education. Even in countries that, in many respects, departed quite radically from their colonial past, values were cherished that were immediately derived from the university system of the former colonial power. Although the conditions in these countries required a more innovative approach, there was often great hesistancy to depart from traditional solutions.

For these countries the absence of truly innovative experiments in Europe and North America certainly was a factor of some importance in the adherence to the well known, to the traditional.

In this paper, I have rather indiscriminately used the terms "university", "medical school", and "medical faculty" as if they indicate more or less identical institutions.

48

On a global basis that is, of course, hardly permissible. In important parts of the world, in particular in a number of socialist countries, the education of doctors is the responsibility of the health care system. Research is the province of universities. The resulting divergence is a factor that can lead to rigidity in the health care system.

The McMaster Concept of Health Professional Education

All the factors mentioned make it difficult to achieve a close collaboration between education, research, and community-based service, the hallmark of a health sciences network. It requires the input of an educational institution which has a clear philosophy that describes its goals in the three areas indicated: the education of doctors; the research it will pursue; and the development of health services it thinks desirable. Such a clear philosophy can be implemented only when management is capable of harnessing the work in the three areas. McMaster was based on such a unified concept. Universities, or medical faculties, or medical schools that wish to pursue a similar course should consider how far their stated goals and their management structure compare to this unified concept.

In the years when the McMaster health sciences program was conceived, medical education all over the world showed signs of unrest. Some of it was generated close to this place, in Buffalo. In these years Miller, Abrahamson, Jason and Rosinsky started their pioneering activities in medical education development. In Europe the British Association for Medical Education gave stimuli in the same direction. Fülop and Miller took a leading role in the development of a global WHO (World Health Organization) teacher training program that stimulated interest in the application of modern educational concepts to the education of health professionals. All over the world the effects of that program can be traced. The development of medical education at McMaster University took its own course, distinct in many respects from the pioneering activities indicated above.

I do not feel qualified to discuss the relationship of all these pioneering activities with the trends and developments in educational psychology and sociology in the same era.

Personally, I had the fortune to work with Jason in Michigan State University. The work at OMERAD (Office for Medical Education Research and Development) profited highly from a close collaboration with a diversity of scientists from fields like educational psychology and sociology. This created a very stimulating and productive environment for innovative work in the teaching of medicine in keeping with current educational science. The educational philosophy that became the basis of the developments at McMaster not only showed a clear perception of what went on in educational science, but represented advanced thinking on the development of health care. The educational concept chosen was in harmony with the requirements of the health care concept.

The McMaster concept presented logical solutions for the major problems that faced medical education, in the sixties, in the seventies and in the eighties.

Four major problem areas exist. They are:

1. Expansion of knowledge that may be useful for medical care.
2. Fragmentation of this knowledge.
3. Lack of relevance of medical education.
4. Rapid changes in medical care and health requirements.

Expansion of knowledge. There is much more knowledge available in the world than we actually use in our efforts to help the sick and to prevent disease. The student's main task is to develop himself into a self-learner who can, for the rest of his professional life, resist the temptation to assume that what he knows at any given moment can offer the best solutions for the problems he is trying to deal with.

Knowledge is accumulating and aging very rapidly. Modern communication technology makes access to this rapidly growing body of knowledge easy in principle; the skills needed to become proficient in "how to look up" and "how to use" are crucially important, and should be very clearly reflected in the curriculum of any medical school.

Only then will "...the self-learning process become a leading objective of ...(an) educational program". The last words, of course, are from Moshe Prywes. It is impossible to discuss medical education without citing some of his wise and visionary published work.

Fragmentation. Much of the knowledge of potential importance for health, health care and medical care is generated by scientists working in the context of disciplines that have often no clear and direct relationship with medical care. Unfortunately, in many universities, the prevailing systems of financing research and of rewarding faculty and staff have emphasized discipline-based research. The same is true for the contributions to the medical curriculum asked from the scientists.

John Evans was not only keenly aware of the problems that resulted from this situation for the development of good medical education; he clearly indicated the need for organizing a medical school so that its objectives in education, research and service could be achieved with a minimum of internal conflict. What he logically thought out appeared to have been invented in industry too: "matrix management."

I bring this concept forward at this place, because I think that the logical solution for the two problem areas mentioned cannot be implemented. In many universities, the organization and the value system conflict with the logical solution. That solution, of course, is "problem-based learning". Flexner already indicated this, in slightly different terms. I shall come back to that later.

At this point, I would like to say that evidence is accumulating that a curriculum based upon the concept of "problem-based learning" offers the best solution to all four problem areas that we are discussing.

The resistance experienced in its implementation has to do with the organizational structure of the educational institute and with vested interests. There are hardly arguments against this concept that can be based upon the outcome of educational research.

51

Relevance. In academic circles the word "relevance" is met with reactions that vary from polite disapproval to outright aggression. There is no doubt that the word has become slightly overworked. It has been misused for many non-scientific or anti-scientific purposes. There are many compelling reasons, however, to bring it up again. In countries all over the world, students assert that their education has assisted them in becoming adequate practitioners in the field of their choice. The demands of health care vary from country to country, because of evolving problems attributable to industrial societies. The traditional training of the doctor no longer offers the best solution to the problems of health and health care of many countries. Primary care in a major part of the world demands an input from the medical professionals taking part in it for which the traditional medical curriculum does not provide.

The McMaster experiment proceeded from a unified concept of teaching and care requirements: a curriculum based upon the health and health care problems that for qualitative and quantitative reasons are important in the region in which the student will work after graduation. Problem-based learning, the concept that seemed logical in the face of increasing expansion and fragmentation of knowledge, provided the best answer in this context as well. Its realization required that research should be directed toward problems of health and disease in the region where the faculty operated. Epidemiology, the study of environmental factors, and the study of the functioning of service systems are areas that provide essential input for this type of curriculum development. Active student participation in this research can speed up the responsiveness of the cybernetic cycle. The study of medical decision-making is of equal importance.

Medical decision-making is a mixture of action based upon empirical data; of tradition; and of action based upon logical conclusions that can be drawn on the basis of data, collected through scientific methods. In fact, in medical education these distinctions are often not clearly made. Problem-based learning can help students in making these

52

distinctions. It will help define areas of great uncertainty. It can contribute to the reduction of these areas. It can help the student develop an atttitude of acceptance of the inevitable uncertainties he has to live with. It can help him to deal with these situations. What is required is, of course, a willingness of teachers to address themselves to the development of knowledge about medical decision-making. The faculty should develop research programs in this area.

It is clear that the three important problem areas discussed so far potentially can be better dealt with through a problem-based learning approach. It is equally clear that there is great hesitancy to adopt this approach. Both in countries that set up their first training of doctors and in countries with a long tradition of university education, there is resistance, often strong resistance.

One element in that resistance is an apparent lack of intellectual respectability of problem-based learning. Often this is confused with types of problem-solving based largely on pattern recognition. The learning process is thought to be limited to the recognition of patterns and to the acquisition of knowledge about practical solutions. In proper problem-based learning the focus should be on the scientific exercise of the application of knowledge, drawn from a rich variety of disciplines to the logical solution of a problem. After analyzing the problem properly, the student has to work out strategies for its solution.

In addition, considerable effort should be spent on a proper evaluation of the quality of the solution. The development of a problem-based curriculum is therefore a rather high-level intellectual exercise that requires the collaboration of teachers with different scientific backgrounds. There is evidence, in slowly increasing amounts, that the learning that results can be highly relevant to the field of application and of commendable intellectual and social respectability.

Unfortunately, the few universities that have committed themselves to this approach to university education have to face all the work required to develop and improve their curricula, while they are faced at the same time with the task of carrying out the research into its usefulness and effectiveness. Given these conditions, one has to admire the progress that has already been made. A good many critics forget that they themselves often continue their educational activities on the unproven assumption that the traditional curriculum provides the desired results. This saves them the energy needed for change and the energy needed for the evaluation of change!

Changes. The needs for medical care and therefore the demands made on its key professionals vary widely. There is a close relationship between the conditions under which human beings live and the disease problems they develop. We know diseases of poverty and disease of affluence.

In the last decade it has been shown that properly directed medical care can improve life expectancy and quality of life in poor countries more rapidly than historical studies in the industrial world suggested to be possible. In these countries, there is in particular a real need for an adaptable, flexible medical care system.

Is the health sciences network better capable of such adaptation? Does the educational approach as chosen by McMaster increase the adaptability of medical care? The relationship between medical education and medical care has been a concern, in varying degrees, throughout history.

Let me cite one example: The leading role of Boerhaave in medical education does not need be brought forward in this audience. One of his contributions was the revival of bedside teaching. Less well known is the specific way in which the communal authorities of Leiden and the curators of the university tried to contribute to the development of a health sciences network. Bedside teaching took place in the Caecilia Hospital. Boerhaave walked every Wednesday from the university to this hospital. The town physicians of Leiden were instructed to accompany him on this walk and discuss their problems with Boerhaave. The curators saw the importance for Boerhaave's teaching of feedback of this type!

After Boerhaave's bedside teaching in the Caecilia hospital, the role of the hospital as a proper environment for the teaching of practical medicine became firmly entrenched. The role of hospital care in the system of medical care changed profoundly, in particular in the last decades. The result is well known in many countries.

Medical education became strongly biased toward hospital-based specialized medical care, neglecting other areas. Universities and medical schools contributed strongly to the development of advanced, specialized medical care. They did not contribute systematically to the overall development of health care and medical care. The model of hospital-based, specialist-centred medical care which they represented and supported influenced the development of health care in less privileged countries in a sometimes detrimental way. Let us consider for a moment the requirements of medical care as they were listed in a recent publication of Taba, the regional director of the Eastern-Mediterranean region of WHO, the man who stimulated important developments in health care in the Middle East.

TABLE II

```
8 essentials elements of

PRIMARY HEALTH CARE          food supply - nutrition
                             safe water and sanitation
                             maternal-child health
                             immunization
                             prevention, control local diseases
                             treatment common disease, injury
                             health education
                             drug provision
a.h. Taba, m.d.
   the learner 7-4, 1979
```

It is clear that many traditional curricula do not contribute very much to these requirements. We have already discussed reasons why problem-based learning fed by the appropriate research can help in improving the relevance of the learning process.

It can help in achieving the important objectives in primary care listed by Taba. The educational process should then, however, be based in the community rather than in the hospital.

Conditions for Community-based Teaching

I would like to spend a few moments on some of the conditions that need to be met before practical teaching can be moved out into the community. Attention should be given to the preparation of community-based teachers for their teaching role and to the quality of the learning environment they provide.

Training. Experience in teacher training, teacher preparation, is rapidly mounting. Given a practitioner whose working conditions permit him to spend time on teaching, it is clear that he can benefit from teacher training, and that properly prepared he will contribute to the learning process just as well as any faculty member. In fact, the non-university based practitioner often takes a greater interest in teaching and finds it intellectually and emotionally more rewarding than his academic colleagues.

Quality of Care. In a health sciences network that is operating properly, there should be good information available on the level of quality that is achieved in different settings of medical care in the community. The presence of students generally enhances the quality of care. An argument against community-based clinical teaching that is often heard is the possible negative effect of exposure to substandard medicine. This argument, in my opinion, is not well founded. There is little evidence that supports the statement that a student will lower his personal standards when confronted with poor medicine, provided of course his previous learning experiences stimulated the development of these standards, and provided there are formal opportunities for discussion of practice experience with teachers and peers.

Consistency. The problem that appears to be more difficult to solve is the important divergence that can exist between the health care concept on which the university bases its teaching and the actual practice of health care. If the student is urged to prepare himself for a role in medical care that is different from the actual roles played by community physicians, then conflict may result. If the university wishes to promote a problem- and patient-centred form of medical care, then an internship or residency in a strongly specialist-centred system can be unproductive and damaging for the learning process.

Control. In the health sciences network, it is important from the educational point of view and from the point of view of health care development that the educational institution has some degree of control over elements of the service system. This is not a veiled effort to bring back the single ivory tower situation. Rather, we need opportunities to develop several model farms. I indicate the need to investigate the amount of control the university needs to achieve its education and service objectives in different health care settings. If medical care delivery is badly organized or is not up to the standards that are desirable from the educational and health service point of view, then mechanisms should be present that can implement change, however slow that change may be.

If the university is not in a position to promote change in community health care, then it cannot achieve some of the goals that are characteristic for its role in a health sciences network. The ivory tower was not compatible with that role; too little control can be just as bad. A careful evaluation of these aspects in the different experiments that are underway may help define the organizational conditions that need to be met. This is of particular importance for countries that are developing care systems from scratch, knowing that the problems they have to take care of may undergo rather rapid change. The health sciences network should, in these conditions, be capable of producing a succession of solutions for health care delivery with the different educational programs and flexible practice settings needed for their implementation. The important matter of control over health care and medical care, of course, is determined by the prevailing system in the country in which education takes place.

With Milton Terris, I would like to distinguish three different systems for the financing of medical care and, therefore, for its control:

1) Public assistance
2) Health insurance
3) National health service

A true systems approach theoretically can best be achieved if medical care is being delivered under the conditions of a national health service. One finds these conditions mainly in socialist countries. In some of these countries, however, research is the exclusive task of universities that operate rather remote from the system of health care. Comparable control is possible in those countries where medical care delivery is done through public assistance, the problem there being lack of finances. In the industrialized world, in many countries, we try to run medical care with individual medical entrepreneurs, modifying inequality of access through different forms of insurance.

The proper operation of a health sciences network will mainly be determined by the political decisions that have been taken about medical care development. The health sciences network can, however, indicate potential alternatives to the politicians based upon intimate knowledge of the medical problems that have to be dealt with, the profiles of personnel available, and other, cultural and organizational, factors that can determine the potential of a health sciences network. Ideally politics should be strongly influenced by the vision and expertise that emanate from such a network.

Some Unresolved Issues

Departures from traditional education such as problem-based learning may be more acceptable to some students than to others. The true systems approach to health and health care as it ideally develops in a health sciences network should make it possible to indicate rather easily the desirable profiles of the professionals needed to run it. Adaptability to the requirements of the learning process and capability for future roles should, according to some, be the target of a selection process that helps choose the right students for the system.

In my own country, there is no legal basis for selection of students that apply for admission to university. They have a constitutional right of entry if they have the necessary academic qualifications. Emergency legislation was created when massive numbers of students that entered university threatened to disrupt university education. The admissible number is selected by lottery with some weighting for high marks in the final high school examination.

The Maastricht experience so far suggests that students so selected are with very few exceptions capable of meeting the demands of problem-based learning in a setting that emphasizes self-learning. It is questionable if selection procedures exist that would make it possible to determine which students whould make the best doctors in the system.

Research suggests that selection procedures can possibly improve the efficiency of education. It is difficult to rule out, however, the influence of factors like teacher attitude, curriculum design, design and use of evaluation procedures, curriculum flexibility, and priority given to education within an institution, factors that equally favour efficiency and effectiveness. The most efficient educational institutions appear to show, in addition to selective admission procedures, a very positive combination of these variables.

In a health sciences network that operates on the basis of common goals for education and health care and in which student education, specialist training and continuing education are well integrated, it may be possible to develop in the long run some selection criteria. It may be equally possible that such a perfect education environment produces the desired results without a need to implement selective admission.

The development and implementation of problem-based learning, with extensive use of community-based health care, is very demanding of teaching staff. Teaching should rank high in their value system. Interest will wane if the reward system does not properly reward good contributions to education. To achieve this it is necessary to have criteria for the proper judgment of the value of contributions to education. Faculty evaluation will only succeed if reasonable objective measurements of educational activity can be achieved. In most faculties, adequate methodology for these measurements is not available.

New approaches to health care and to education for the health sciences require proper institutional evaluation. I have indicated already the problems that result when the heavy workload brought about by implementation of a new program is worsened by the need to spend energy on the development of proper program evaluation. The workload can sometimes be reduced by inter-institutional collaboration leading to a division of tasks and to an intensive exchange of information. This may be an important task for the network recently initiated by the World Health Organization.

In my experience, the use of external observers is extremely valuable for the provision of the feedback that is needed to steer an innovative course. In Maastricht, the material provided by the permanent external review committee chaired by Hilliard Jason and a series of reports written by critical observers like George Miller, Vic Neufeld and Baghman Joorabchi proved to be invaluable.

Objective measurement of output cannot be done in this way, however. The magnitude of the task of development of the proper tools and the execution of the research puts it beyond the capacity of the average medical faculty, particularly when the budget is light. Collaboration can, as indicated, be of help. Outside funding of collaborative research on the results of ongoing experiments will have to be found so that we will be capable of making well-founded statements on the advantages and disadvantages of problem-based learning in the setting of the health sciences network.

For those who have been actively engaged in this work, there is little doubt about its exciting potential. The enthusiasm of John Evans at the present time is shared by many. The foundation of the McMaster Faculty of Health Sciences was the beginning of a new era in medical education!

The McMASTER M.D. PROGRAM

BASIC PREMISES AND CURRICULUM

by WILLIAM SPAULDING, M.D.
Professor, Department of Medicine, Faculty of Health Sciences
McMaster University
Hamilton, Ontario, Canada

The 1950's and 1960's were times of unusual dissatisfaction with medical education. Critics ranged from disgruntled medical students to disenchanted patients and to the new breed of medical educators led by George Miller.

The graduates of medical schools at that time were seen by some as too conservative, lacking in imagination and enterprise, too committed to technology, and not committed enough to humanism. Others felt that medical students came from overly circumscribed educational backgrounds typified by tightly constructed pre-medical courses, spent too long at their undergraduate and graduate education before beginning to serve the community, were insensitive to community needs, and were too materialistic.

The medical schools themselves were criticized for placing too much emphasis on teaching and too little on learning. Rewards went to the research achievements of faculty, and little attention was paid to good teaching. Many schools had rigid departmental organizations which placed too much power in the hands of entrenched chairmen and deprived enthusiastic young faculty of the opportunity to innovate in education. It was felt there was an over-emphasis on the minutiae of basic biological sciences and too little emphasis on behavioural and community issues. Students were rewarded for cramming facts to achieve high marks on examinations in a highly competitive system, while little attention was paid to their personal qualities such as intellectual curiosity and compassion.

All these influences were at work in 1966 when John Evans asked myself, Jim Anderson, Fraser Mustard and Bill Walsh to form an education

committee to construct a curriculum. After preliminary discussion,
Dr. Evans sketched a three-year curriculum with four phases, no courses,
and considerable time for electives. He gave the four of us maximum
freedom to work out an educational approach and develop the curriculum in
detail.

All of us realized we had a remarkable opportunity to innovate and
experiment, and none of us wanted to stand pat or play it safe; we were
eager to try out very different approaches to what we ourselves had
experienced and see whether these approaches would mould a better medical
graduate.

The backgrounds of the early planners had certain similarities.
John Evans and three out of four on the committee were all graduates of
the University of Toronto, while the fourth, Bill Walsh, had graduated
from the University of Western Ontario and taken postgraduate training in
Toronto. Anderson had taught anatomy and anthropology and been deeply
involved in community problems of adolescents; Mustard, an experimental
pathologist, had concentrated on research in thrombosis, and had been
involved in graduate education and the general pathology course at the
University of Toronto. Walsh was a general internist in Hamilton, and I
was a general internist full time in the medical school in Toronto. We
all knew each other and had had similar experience as medical students:
in general, three years of premedical and preclinical science lectures
and laboratories, then three years of increasing bedside and outpatient
involvements. This undoubtedly helped us to agree quickly on certain
changes to be introduced. The twelve premises on which the M.D. Program
was based and the ways in which these premises were expressed in the
curriculum and admission requirements are listed in the Appendices A and
B.

The single most important objective was to graduate students who
would, throughout their working life, be able to solve problems and learn
effectively on their own. Because it was obvious that during the
lifetime of each graduate, knowledge would have to be renewed continually
and applied to a variety of problems - some of which could not even be

foreseen – we wished to maximize learning and minimize teaching. The graduate MUST know how to learn, but the sources of most of the teaching would be his or her patients and the local learning materials available for study. As much as possible, students had to be responsible for their own education. The job of faculty was to help students to learn effectively and extensively.

For self-learning, students needed to have most of their time available to use as they wished. Only a minimum was to be taken up by lectures or other scheduled teaching sessions. (Early on, the guideline was that only an hour a day should be scheduled for didactic sessions such as lectures or laboratory exercises.) Because students vary considerably in their styles of learning, learning resources had to be available in a variety of media, much beyond the usual library collection of books and journals. An organization for learning resources was begun well before the medical school opened. All faculty were encouraged to produce slide/tape shows for study by students in a specially equipped room, and several hundred were available when the first students came in 1969. A slide/tape display unit was designed, and purchased in what proved to be unnecessarily large numbers. Faculty produced videotapes; pathological specimens were prepared and described. These extensive learning resources were catalogued as part of the library collection, with a single catalogue system identifying for the learner all the materials available for study.

We decided that virtually the entire curriculum should be based on a series of biomedical problems. In a sense, the biomedical problems became the core curriculum and formed the backbone of the course up until the clinical clerkship. From that point on, patients for whom clerks were responsible provided real-life problems as a basis for learning. We felt that if problem topics were well chosen, the selection of appropriate program content would follow automatically. Well-selected and well-prepared problems could lead the student into those areas of study thought to be important. If, for example, the problem topic was:

64

"How does a person respond to a severe burn?", the content and resources
should include water, electrolyte and protein changes, surface barriers
to infection, tissue healing, and psychological responses to pain,
disfigurement, prolonged hospital care and disability. In addition to
current references, there should be knowledgeable people to whom the
student could turn for advice, perhaps best encountered in a burn unit.

In most of the problems, basic science and clinical medicine were
interwoven to help students learn a scientific approach to problems. The
advantage of a small tutorial group as the basic unit for teaching and
learing was so apparent that we put the students and faculty together in
groups of five students to one tutor. Students who had been selected
from a variety of educational and work backgrounds could help to teach
each other during tutorials, those with science backgrounds learning from
those with backgrounds in the humanities, and vice versa. The tutor
could guide the learning and help the students improve their ability to
deal with biomedical problems. During tutorials, interaction between
members would become a feature, and students and tutor could identify
what constitutes favourable dynamics and what constitutes inhibiting
behaviour. One of the objectives was to have both students and faculty
learn to function effectively in groups, and for this the tutorial
provided a favourable milieu. In a small group, faculty and students
would become well acquainted, and much informal guidance could ensue.
The group approach has been used more formally to enhance interviewing
skills and examine human behaviour.

Having in mind the multiplicity of problems which confront research
workers, practitioners and community organizers, we felt that a mix of
different types of people should be admitted to the medical school.
Accordingly, admission requirements were drawn up to encourage students
from non-science university backgrounds to apply. This decision greatly
enlarged our pool of applicants, because many students were only eligible
to apply to McMaster. An elaborate admission process, with many people
involved in selection and interviewing, has resulted from the endeavour

to stress the personal qualities of students as well as their academic backgrounds and achievements.

By the time students were selected for admission to medical school, we felt they had demonstrated that they were able learners. To avoid emphasis on high marks and class standing, the usual examination system was not employed in evaluation, and no marks or class standings were awarded. No medals, scholarships or other financial supports were awarded for academic achievement; instead financial need was the prime criterion for monetary assistance.

We felt that students should have liberal opportunities to explore fields of their own choosing in their elective time. To this end, blocks of elective time totalling 26 weeks out of the span of 124 weeks were allocated. Initially, we agreed that if a student was performing satisfactorily and wanted to go and lie on a beach in the sun for four weeks, that could be an acceptable elective. We do, however, require an elective supervisor, and so far no students have persuaded anyone to supervise their sunbathing! The electives provide a welcome change from the intensity of a three-year course in which the longest holiday is a month in the summer.

Since the content of medical knowledge is changing rapidly, with new disciplines emerging, we aimed for maximum flexibility to allow frequent and, if necessary, drastic changes to be built into the curriculum. We wanted to involve as many faculty as possible in planning and working with medical students, and "faculty" included a large number of community practitioners. Rather than develop a vertical, pyramidal hierarchy where the chairman of each department has control over a segment of time during the course, we designated small groups of faculty to plan each portion of the curriculum. Because the units and biomedical problem topics themselves often involved more than one academic discipline, the small groups nearly always contained a mix of faculty from different departments. In the early planning, we deliberately avoided giving any major responsibility to a departmental chairman in order to avoid inhibiting contributions from junior faculty members by a show of rank. In fact, we had several planning groups where we appointed a very junior person as the chairman, with a very senior departmental chairman sitting as a member of the group. Each phase and each unit within a phase had a chief planner, with a small group of faculty and students responsible for modifications and improvements.

In summary, the McMaster medical program incorporated a number of major innovations. The most unique was the development of a series of biomedical problems as a framework for learning the content of a medical course and for developing skills in the solution of problems. The use of tutorial groups to facilitate learning was another. Involvement of many staff and students in curriculum development and revision with no control of the curriculum by departments (except in the clerkship) was also an innovation, and avoidance of class standings and prizes for academic achievement was, and still is, unusual.

THE McMASTER M.D. PROGRAM

BASIC PREMISES AND CURRICULUM: FROM A STUDENT'S POINT OF VIEW

by Lawrence Paszat, M.D.
Student in the Undergraduate M.D. Program, Class of 1980
at the time of the 10th Anniversary Conference

Dr. William Spaulding stated the premise that doctors with diverse attitudes and backgrounds are needed. McMaster does indeed admit students from a very wide spectrum of backgrounds.

I entered the M.D. Program at age 23, having previously completed a B.A. at Victoria College in the University of Toronto. My field of study was ancient middle eastern languages and literature. I had also worked part time in suburban Toronto directing recreational programs for children and adults with special needs and handicaps.

Many McMaster students bring such diversity to medicine. In my first tutorial group there was a nurse, a cytogeneticist, a social worker and a biologist. Each of us brought a unique and valuable perspective, including research in basic science, involvement with family crises and poverty, and interest in women's liberation. It was a very rich and mind-expanding experience for me. Acquiring a broader outlook and undertanding a little bit of the contributions of varied professions was an important part of my education.

This diversity really cannot be quantified; however, the following facts do confirm that McMaster draws its students from many backgrounds. Most of the data to follow are to be found in Appendices A and B.

Data

Fully 1/3 of the students are age 26 or older on admission and 9 percent have been over age 31. However, only one McMaster undergraduate had become a grandparent prior to graduation.

While 35 percent of the cumulative total of McMaster graduates are women, this increases yearly. About 45 percent of the class graduating in May, 1980 were female. Fifty-five percent of the class admitted in September, 1979 were women.

Almost the entire student population completed an undergraduate degree prior to admission. About 4 percent of entering students have earned doctorates, and a total of 28 percent have one or more postgraduate degrees.

Less than 60 percent of McMaster students pursued degrees in natural sciences prior to medical school. Ten percent of entering students have previously trained in other health care professions. One-third of the students come from non-natural-science, non-health-science backgrounds.

Most (about 75 percent) of the entering students have undergraduate grade point averages greater than 3.0 on the 0-4 scale, with 27.5 percent of the class being greater than 3.5. If the 25 percent with grade point averages of less than 3.0 have raised some eyebrows, then Dr. Robert Issenman's remarks on statistics on McMaster graduates will be of considerable interest.

What Really Happens in the M.D. Program at McMaster?

The class is divided into groups of five. These groups change every ten weeks. Each group is assigned a tutor from the faculty and a clinical skills supervisor.

At the beginning of each section, the tutor and the group receive booklets which outline the learning objectives for the particular phase or part-phase. These booklets also list suggested printed and audio-visual instruction material. Usually there is a collection of biomedical problems, including data from history and physical examination and reports from the investigation.

The group will meet with the tutor two or three times weekly. The agenda for these tutorial meetings is planned by the students. With the learning objective in view, the students select biomedical problems for consideration and study. The objectives of the M.D. Program are met in this deliberate fashion.

From time to time the group members may work quite closely with each other outside of the formal tutorial times. Often each member of the group will have an individual plan of attack on a biomedical problem, with the group assembling to pool resources later in the tutorial session.

Can a linguist, who does not know what a cell is, solve a biomedical problem in carbohydrate metabolism along with the other students in his group? Can a group of five medical students, whose tutor is a psychiatrist, learn rheumatology? The answer to both questions is "yes", with several provisions.

First, tutors do not have primarily a didactic role. The tutors' main functions are to assist the group in working efficiently, to help the group identify problems and deficiencies, and to help the group to select appropriate resources to rectify the difficulties, whether in the academic area or in group function.

Second, the primary method of acquiring knowledge is not the tutorial meeting. There is a very large collection of audio-visual instruction materials which have been prepared by the faculty. There is also an excellent library which includes multiple copies of reprinted articles as well as suggested monographs. Also, in some sections of the M.D. Program, one or two didactic sessions daily may be offered by specialists in the relevant fields. Therefore, having a psychiatrist or an obstetrician as a tutor does not impede our learning of rheumatology.

Third, and equally important, are the learning skills of the students. The development of the problem-solving approach to biomedical problems, the refinement of self-directed learning, and the ability to learn from and share with one's peers enable the linguist who is studying medicine at McMaster to deal with the problem in carbohydrate metabolism.

How is the Course Laid Out?

The M.D. Program involves thirty-one months of study, spread over three years. It is divided into several unequal blocks of time.

During the first ten weeks new students are introduced to the McMaster setting and style of education. At this time, students learn

70

how to learn medicine with four other students and a tutor, and how to use efficiently the array of resources available for learning.

Those of us who did not have academic backgrounds in natural sciences began a rapid assimilation of key concepts in cell biology and biochemistry. We were assisted by designated faculty, and to a greater extent by fellow students. The approach used was to tackle the concepts of cell biology and biochemistry which were relevant to whatever biomedical problem we were trying to solve together as a group of five. Indeed, this is the style in which all academic basic medical sciences are incorporated into the M.D. Program.

The development of interviewing ability and clinical skills begins in Phase 1. In continues formally until the clerkship year. The biomedical problem for consideration in a tutorial session was sometimes a patient whom my group had interviewed and examined. It was a real advantage to begin learning basic medical sciences and clinical skills simultaneously. It was very exciting to learn the names and location and function of the heart valves, and to hear "S1" and "S2" for the first time on the very same afternoon. Pulmonary mechanics were a bit easier to grasp when explained during a demonstration of the examination of the chest. Perhaps the significance of quite a bit of the physiology was more easily grasped when correlated to a patient.

At the beginning of Phase 1 each student is assigned to a member of the faculty who will be his or her advisor throughout the Program. Students meet with their advisors once every four to eight weeks to discuss general progress and to formulate goals. Most find that the advisor becomes a friend as well. My own advisor was able to provide helpful observations about evaluations I had received. He was also very helpful when I was planning my elective time and when I was making plans to study areas in which I was very interested, or in which I felt lacking.

It is quite common for individual students or groups of students to plan to pursue areas of interest such as nutrition, human sexuality, or

71

radiology at a more intensive level. It is possible to devote one or two half-days weekly to such interests, concurrently with the phases of the M.D. Program. At various times I spent such time in emergency medicine, pharmacology, and infectious diseases.

Phase II is a very intensive eleven-week period of self-directed learning and problem-solving based on simulated and real clinical problems. Basic normal and pathologic mechanisms are studied intensively. The style of small group tutorials and clinical and interviewing skills development continues.

Phase II is followed by a four-week block of elective time. Each student plans the time and makes all necessary arrangements, which include finding a supervisor. At this early time some select clinical experience. Others spend time in microbiology or pathology labs as I did. The possibilities for elective topics are endless.

Forty of the next fifty-two weeks comprise Phase III. Each body system is studied in turn. The systems are clustered into ten-week units. The problem-solving approach is applied throughout. Through self-directed learning, appropriate aspects of anatomy, physiology, pathology and pharmacology are applied to biomedical problems. Clinical experience pertinent to the system under study is usually available.

There is a five-week summer holiday and a one-week Christmas break during Phase III.

After the first three units, there is a six-week block of elective time. Again, each individual student must write his own ticket. Many more choose clinical experiences during this elective. Many travel abroad.

There are a great many places to which McMaster students have travelled for electives. My time was spent at an exceptionally under-serviced rural hospital in the West Indies. I was supervised much less than I had hoped, but problem-solving and self-directed learning skills made the time one of the most valuable exercises during my degree. This elective also stimulated an interest in health care in developing

72

situations. As a result, I returned to that hospital during one of my clerkship electives, and I am planning a brief third visit immediately after graduation in May of this year (1980).

Phase IV is the clinical clerkship year. In addition to thirty-two weeks in the inpatient and outpatient services, there are sixteen weeks of elective time, and four weeks of holidays. In addition to my return elective to the West Indies, during my clerkship I did electives in orthopedics, ophthalmology, and nephrology. This phase of the M.D. Program at McMaster probably differs least from other medical schools. However, tutorial groups still have a role and the methods and purposes are unchanged. One of the highlights of my clerkship was the significant amount of time that I was able to spend in outpatient settings during pediatrics, obstetrics and gynecology, internal medicine, and general surgery.

Evaluation in the M.D. Program is based on daily contact with faculty and peers in the tutorial meetings, and during Phase IV by direct supervision on the wards. There are also specific evaluation procedures such as written essays on biomedical problems, using a problem-solving approach, and other time-limited exercises to assess problem-solving and self-directed learning skills. I found that the comments I received enabled me to make changes in my approach, unlike the letter grades without comments which I had received for my work during my B.A. Evaluation is formalized by completion of the summary statement of student learning progress, at the end of each unit or phase. This is done by the tutor, usually in collaboration with the student and his or her peers.

M.D. students are members of most of the planning committees of the medical school. The McMaster Medical Student Society holds annual elections for these positions. I was a student member of the M.D. Education Committee during my clerkship. Along with several other students, I attended a one-day Retreat at which broad issues concerning the medical school were discussed. I am also part of a committee which met in September, 1979 to plan this afternoon's meeting.

73

What are the Sore Spots for a Student in this M.D. Program?

Anxiety is a byword among students and faculty, especially in the first three phases. It is not a major problem for all students. At times the anxiety appears to be caused by real or perceived deficits in knowledge, by the absence of a comprehensive and definite syllabus, and by the amount of initiative demanded of students in directing their own learning. Another source of anxiety is the evaluation process. Some students anticipate evaluation of progress and knowledge with apprehension, because there is no core content to be mastered for reiteration. Some worry that an individual faculty person might interpret objectives and parameters of evaluation at a level much more demanding than expected by most evaluators.

At some time during medical school, most students find themselves in a tutorial group that is not functioning smoothly. There may be difficulties between students, or the tutor may have radically different views about style, approach and priorities than those of the students. The resolution of such conflict inevitably consumes emotional energy. While unpleasant, it is an opportunity to learn how to handle disputes and stresses.

Conclusions

In order to summarize my experience of studying medicine at McMaster, I would like to list what I perceived my responsibilities as a student to be:

1. To plan my own education in keeping with the general goals of the M.D. Program and the specific objectives of each phase, and to learn medicine by rigorously carrying out these plans.

2. To evaluate my progress.

3. To contribute to the education and evaluation of my peers.

4. To evaluate my teachers.

5. To assist in some aspects of the planning of the M.D. Program.

6. To be involved in patient care during the clerkship year.

It has not been easy to undertake this thirty-one month program. Nevertheless it has been very exciting, and skills have been acquired which will be useful throughout my career, and which I expect will stand me in good stead during postgraduate training.

THE McMASTER M.D. PROGRAM

BASIC PREMISES AND CURRICULUM: THE VIEWPOINT OF A GRADUATE

by Robert Issenman, M.D.
Pediatric gastroenterologist and part-time member
of the Department of Pediatrics, Faculty of Health Sciences
McMaster University
Hamilton, Ontario, Canada

I graduated from McMaster Medical School in 1973. My previous background was an honours B.A. in political science, one year of law school, and a smattering of C's and B's in pre-med science courses. To a raw graduate of McMaster, an experimental medical school, the greeting of new interns at the Montreal Children's Hospital brought many fears.

The McMaster graduates certainly were different as entering medical students. Our education has been unorthodox. I wondered whether we really were as different by the time we graduated.

We had come with unusual prior qualifications and had been educated without lectures and spent hours in small group tutorials. We had passed without exams. I wondered whether we were qualified.

We had been subjected to an early clinical exposure, a curriculum stressing behavioural aspects and an integrated perspective. Were we in some ways better qualified? Qualified or not, would we be accepted by colleagues, by patients and finally by licensing boards and funding agencies? Many others had the same questions and watched. Now, ten years after having entered medical school, some of the answers are available with the help of statistics compiled by Dr. Christel Woodward as part of an ongoing tracking of graduates.

On the first attempt, 88 percent of our class passed the L.M.C.C., the qualifying examination allowing license ability. This rate was comparable to other medical schools, in many of which the curriculum is more closely tied to preparation for the licencing examinations. In subsequent years, the pass rate on the L.M.C.C. has continued at 92 percent.

Certainly we were accepted into internships without hesitation. In the first two years 86 percent received their first choice in a national matching program. I wondered whether this was done more to test our mettle than as a statement of confidence in us. Nevertheless, the trend has continued. Yearly, 75 percent of graduates achieve their first choice on the matching program, compared to a national average of 66 percent of graduates across the country participating in the national match. In my class, 50 percent selected for primary care programs rather than specialty training. This was of interest because many thought the original McMaster program had emphasized preparation for primary care. I elected a straight internship in pediatrics and went to the Montreal Children's Hospital. Some 47 percent of our graduates have similarly specialized with almost 20 percent entering internal medicine.

Recalling the exacting and unusual admission procedures, I recall wondering whether my personal qualities were better than those of my fellow interns. They had been selected largely, it would seem, on the grade point average. Happily, they seemed to possess as many "personal qualities" as I flattered myself with having. It seemed clear that while medical students at most schools were selected without regard to their merit as human beings, those chosen for this competitive residency program had been subjected to a second selection process which emphasized character as well as competence.

As to the competence, this is a quality which the individual is at great disadvantage to self-assess. However, successive classes have reported that they felt as well prepared (or as ill prepared) as their peers, for their role in internship. Of the first four classes surveyed, 24 percent felt better prepared, 63 percent felt equally qualified.

I certainly felt ill at ease when I let my imagination wander to all the diseases that had never been covered in our tutorials. I soon realized that a residency is a very supportive environment in which most of the knowledge is acquired by osmosis. What distinguished me from other interns was that I lacked the clinical panache and confidence which others had acquired during longer and more classical clerkships. On the other hand, I had an excellent background in interviewing techniques and patient management skills. A survey of the first four graduating classes from McMaster reinforced my own impressions. McMaster graduates felt very comfortable in the ambulatory setting dealing with social and emotional problems. They were competent in their ability to problem solve and gather data. They felt well prepared for independent learning. They had real insecurity in their basic science information base. Similarly, they felt weak as to drug effects and comparatively poor in medical emergencies.

In my perspective, I found the subjects that I had taught myself, such as pathology and biochemistry, more serviceable for me in the day-to-day problems than they appeared to be for my internship colleagues, even though these disciplines were not taught as distinct courses. My friends had a more solid grounding in these disciplines but little practice in relating time to their work and learning as clinicians. My understanding of these subjects, while less comprehensive, seemed more useful. However, the main difference seemed that my education had been enjoyable. My friends' perspective on medical school was that it had been a trial. I decided then that the educational system at McMaster had merit even if the results were equal, to the extent that it preserved the pleasure of learning needlessly sacrificed at other institutions.

Looking back, graduates of the program in the first four years valued many of the same aspects to which I alluded: small group tutorials and independent study within a flexible system based on problem-based learning. They enjoyed early patient contact and the faculty commitment. They considered the evaluation system and the lack of definition of core material weaknesses. They uniformly commented on the anxiety level generated, because without exams few students felt they really knew where they stood. At the same time, most considered the anxiety this produced as a useful stimulus to study. The favoured

78

element of the program was the fact that it was shorter. Eighty-two percent of the classes valued the fact that they spent three years in medical school rather than four. This provided a clear appreciation of each element of the course from the opening day. The question of relevance was never as much of an issue at McMaster as it was at other medical schools. There was little questioning of the need to learn the subject matter, only the persistant question about whether there was enough time to cover it all.

Upon finishing two years of pediatric training I elected to move on to Boston. Like many of my peers, these moves were made on the basis of contacts made during internship and residency, rather than the medical school experience. By this time my training at McMaster as an experimental medical school seemed remote. It made little impact on those who interviewed me. They relied almost entirely on personal recommendation of my clinical supervisors during residency years.

Acceptance did not seem to loom as a major problem for graduates of McMaster. Fifty-eight percent of the first four classes went on to complete full residencies. Forty percent have been certified either by the Royal College of Physicians and Surgeons or the College of Family Physicians.

My education at McMaster only emerged as an obstacle for me when I attempted to win a Medical Research Council scholarship. I was turned down for this on the basis that I had no classical undergraduate transcript. This I felt reflected as badly on the Medical Research Council as it did on myself but could have been an irreversible blow to my career, though fortunately I was able to win competitive funding from other sources. More recent graduates have not encountered the same problems, having obtained MRC fellowships and Robert Wood Johnson fellowships.

As a research fellow in Boston, I made the passing acquaintance of dozens of New Zealand white rabbits. I also encountered 20 percent of my class who were at the Harvard Teaching Hospitals doing postgraduate work. In Boston, the absence of a rigorous core curriculum in my undergraduate medical education did not represent a handicap for me, even when I went into the laboratory. It was reasonably easy to acquire laboratory technique. My more conventionally trained colleagues had equal difficulty designing well-controlled experiments, and certainly broke as many pipettes.

Upon completing the Fellowship, I returned to Canada and joined 80 percent of McMaster graduates in the country. Sixty-two percent are in Ontario. Sixteen percent of the graduates from 1972 to 1978 are in the United States. I returned because of the unusual opportunity to practice consultation pediatrics in an urban area, with a close relationship to an academic centre.

The strongest determinants of location for my colleagues were different. The first was the influence of a spouse; the second was high medical need in the area; the third was a preference for a particular urban or rural lifestyle. At this time, about half of the McMaster graduates are in practice. Forty percent are in group practices and 31 percent are in solo practices. Most live in metropolitan cities, and the rest are equally divided between towns, medium-size cities and rural areas.

On assuming practice, I have felt very well prepared. My career seems to require equal measures of what I was taught in residency and what was offered to me in medical school. Of great help has been the strong background in behavioural issues. Less important has been the lack of formal teaching in the basic sciences.

Most surprising was the appreciation that came to me, that my own perspective had gradually but insidiously changed during the years. This fall I was called upon to teach Phase I medical students as an expert tutor in the area of pediatric gastroenterology. As the session progressed, I found myself astounded at the ignorance of some fundamentals displayed by these medical students. I asked myself if it was possible that these individuals, ignorant at that time of the concept of a cell and of the exact relationship of digestive enzymes to the anatomy of the gastrointestinal tract, could ever be transformed into physicians in a short thirty-three month period. I am sure that the same uncertainty plagued my own teachers ten years ago. Perhaps the greatest asset possessed by these medical students is their capacity for growth, and the greatest strength of the medical school curriculum is the encouragement of this indigenous learning potential.

THE McMASTER M.D. PROGRAM

FACTORS IMPORTANT FOR CHANGE

by Ronald McAuley, M.D.

Professor, Department of Family Medicine and Chairman of the
Undergraduate M.D. Program at the time of the 10th Anniversary Conference
Faculty of Health Sciences, McMaster University
Hamilton, Ontario, Canada

Introduction

I had been in general practice in Hamilton when Dr. Bill Walsh asked
me about my interest in the new medical school. The question was a brief
one: What was the part that community physicians might play in the new
school? The result was that four of us joined the school with
Dr. Spaulding as our mentor and set up a Residency Program in Family
Medicine in 1967.

My first involvement with the Undergraduate M.D. Program was in
assisting Dr. Jim Anderson with the planning and implementation of the
first Phase I, which began in 1969 with twenty students.

I then became interested in the process of selecting medical
students, working closely with Dr. Alex Adsett and Dr. John Hamilton, who
subsequently followed Dr. Bill Spaulding as chairmen of the M.D.
Program. After three years as Admissions Chairman, I became the M.D.
Program Chairman in 1975 when Dr. Hamilton completed his term of office.
My observations are provided from this vantage point.

I will focus upon three questions related to change:

- What changes have occurred since the M.D. Program began in 1969?
- What do we need to do better?
- What is our capacity for change?

What Changes Have Occurred Since the M.D. Program Began in 1969?

No major changes have occurred in the M.D. Program since its
inception. The changes I will describe are really refinements that have
occurred as a result of our collective experience in implementing the

basic concepts. Some of the changes are a response to the increase in the number of students and faculty, and some are the results of studies carried out over the years. I have selected ten items which I consider to be important.

1. The Selection of Students for the M.D. Program

After trying out several methods for selecting students in the early 1970's, an approach was adopted which assessed both the academic and personal characteristics of applicants. Emphasis was placed upon characteristics considered important to enable students to achieve the objectives of the M.D. Program, such as problem-solving ability and self-appraisal ability, and characteristics which help them to be the types of physicians that we felt were needed by the community. Another decision was made to ask people from four constituencies to actually do the assessment. Most or all schools have involved faculty, and many have involved students; but we decided to also share the responsibility with the practising medical profession and with the consumers. We asked a variety of community groups to help identify people who could take part in letter-reading and interviewing. Beginning in 1976 it became possible for applicants without university degrees to apply for the M.D. Program. Our first two applicants in this category graduated last year and this year, and they have coped as well as those who had university degrees. In 1981 applicants over the age of thirty will be looked at more carefully, as a result of findings from a recently completed study about the relationship of admission variables to in-course and Medical Council of Canada examination performance.

2. Preliminary Program

In the early years of the M.D. Program a summer course was established for new students lacking university courses in either the behavioral or the biological sciences. The behavioral science program was stopped after one year and the biological science program was discontinued after five years. While the students in the biological program found it helpful in learning the language of science and in

improving problem-solving skills, the decision to discontinue the program
was based upon the principle that help should be provided when, and if,
it is required in order for students to solve biomedical problems.

3.   Phase I

Phase I is designed to assist students with the transition to
problem-based and self-directed learning. With a group of broad health
care problems, such as the "Joseph Smith" problem in Appendix A, students
learn to develop and test out hypotheses, to use a variety of educational
resources, and to assume responsibility for their own learning in a group
setting. Tutors and selected Phase III students provide ongoing
assistance. Resource people in both the biological and behavioral
sciences are available when assistance is needed. The various support
systems provided during Phase I have done much to help students adapt to
the M.D. Program.

4.   Concurrent Phase III

Until 1975 each unit of Phase III was presented once a year.
However, with the increase in class size and the limited learning
resources available, the decision was reached to present each unit four
times during the year. This reduced the number of students in a unit to
twenty-five at a time. While one disadvantage was that planners were
involved on a year round basis, there were distinct advantages to the
students.

5.   Electives

Six and one-half of the thirty-one months of the M.D. Program are
set aside for electives. Over the years, we have continued to see great
diversity in the type of electives and the locations chosen. Faculty has
continued to give support to electives; they are of equal status to the
required phases and units, and graduating students have repeatedly
identified electives as one of the major strengths of the M.D. Program.
Electives are used to explore areas of special interest, and to make up
real or perceived deficiencies. The experience does much to develop

students' maturity and their skills in being self-directed learners, because they are responsible for all aspects of the electives.

6. Excessive Structure

Excessive structure developed in some phases and units with the result that students often had little time for pursuing learning on their own. The biomedical problems were often inadequate as learning stimuli, the necessary resources for biomedical problems were not always readily available, and planners had scheduled many large group sessions, otherwise known as lectures. In some units in the clinical clerkship, that is Phase IV, excessive patient care demands had reduced the time and attention that students could give to achieving the educational objectives of the phase and the M.D. Program. In 1979 the M.D. Education Committee and subsequently the Phase Committees made several changes. In Phase III the number of lectures was reduced by 50 percent, and planners initiated a systematic review of all biomedical problems in their units. In Phase IV the relationship between education and patient care was re-assessed. The decision was reached that patient care, while important, was not the only means for students to achieve the objectives of the phase. This permitted a reduction in the service demands upon students in some units. The chairmen of clinical departments supported this decision.

7. Competence of Tutors

In 1975 the M.D. Program required 150 tutors during the academic year for the three classes. Concern was being expressed about the uneven level of performance of tutors by both students and the M.D. Program planners. This was not surprising, given the lack of experience of many faculty members in the facilitative role required of the tutor. After the problem was reviewed by the M.D. Education Committee, the Health Sciences Education Committee, and Faculty Executive, the following initiatives were taken:

    i)   Workshops were established by the Program for Educational
           Development for the training of tutors. During the

85

two-and-a-half-day workshops, faculty members had repeated
opportunities to practice their skills in recognizing and
dealing with problems of group learning by working with five
students in a simulated tutorial with five colleagues watching
from behind one-way windows. Following each 20-minute session,
self-evaluation was obtained as well as feedback from both the
students and colleagues. You will note the use of the same
basic premises outlined by Dr. Spaulding in the education of
faculty.

(ii)   The system for faculty evaluation was reviewed by the M.D.
Education Committee and students were asked to evaluate their
tutors using the same principles as were used for student
evaluation. An evaluation form was developed which identified
the characteristics to be assessed.

(iii)   Program planners became more involved in the selection,
orientation and monitoring of their tutors.

(iv)   Departmental chairmen emphasized the importance of tutoring
during their annual review with members of their departments.
The tutor evaluation reports had an influence upon
consideration for promotion and tenure.

(v)   Departmental chairmen, deans and educational leaders tutored
each year.

The result of these initiatives was an increase in the number of
skilled tutors. However, there is still need for ongoing effort at
assisting faculty members in improving their effectiveness as tutors.

8.   Student Evaluation

While the principles upon which the evaluation of students is based
have not changed over the years, the task of implementation has proven
difficult. This is not surprising, considering the nature of the task.
Dr. Hilliard Jason commented in a visit in the early 1970's that an
evaluation system in fact did not exist. Accreditation reports have
noted deficiencies in evaluation, and graduating students have repeatedly

86

identified evaluation as a major problem area. During the past five
years we have taken the following incentives:

i) An Objectives Task Group has submitted a comprehensive report
on the M.D. Program objectives and the objectives for the basic
medical science disciplines.

ii) The objectives for the four phases of the M.D. Program have
been or are being revised.

iii) Different methods for evaluating skills such as problem solving
are being developed and tested.

iv) The tutors' reports about student performance in the phases and
units are now being completed on all students. Although still
uneven, more reports each year are recording specific
information about performance in designated areas such as
problem solving, strengths and weaknesses. As a result,
student advisors now possess more information upon which to
base the students' academic transcripts at the end of the M.D.
Program.

v) An evaluation manual prepared by the Evaluation Committee is
currently being reviewed by the M.D. Education Committee.

vi) An effective support group prepares individualized remedial
programs for students receiving "unsatisfactory" evaluations.

Much remains to be done in order for students and faculty to both
give and receive ongoing, honest, constructive criticism.

9. Student Involvement

Student representatives are members on all M.D. program groups,
including search committees for program leaders and boards that consider
students with serious academic problems. Their commitment and
contributions are highly regarded. The students organize the program
each year for preparation for the Medical Council of Canada
examinations. There is now a Medical Student Society and an Alumni
organization. The large number of M.D. Program graduates enrolled in the

various McMaster residency programs play a significant role in the education of students, especially in Phase IV.

10. Followup Studies

Because of the different approach being taken in the education of our medical students, it is important that studies about the graduates are conducted. A computerized data bank has been established which links admissions data with outcome variables such as performance in the M.D. Program, Medical Council of Canada examination results, residency program choices, specialty examination results, and the nature and location of practice. A three-year study of the performance of graduates during their internship year is currently being completed. Feedback is also obtained at regular intervals about the graduates' perceptions about the M.D. Program.

Summaries of these studies are contained in Appendices A and B and detailed reports are available.

What Do We Need to Do Better?

In the recently completed reports by the Task Groups established by Faculty Executive, three areas were identified which require future attention:

1. Evaluation of Students and Faculty

While initiatives have been taken to improve the evaluation systems, there is much that remains to be done. Workshops are needed for planners and tutors to review the evaluation process and the methods for assessing performance of students and recording findings. Based upon the findings from two studies, student advisors need assistance in preparing the transcripts which summarize the reports from tutors and electives supervisors about their students.

Evaluation instruments need to be developed, tested and validated. Students needs assistance in preparing honest reports about the performance of faculty. While some reports by students clearly label strengths and weaknesses of faculty members in various educational roles,

88

there is much room for improvement. Similarly, many planners could provide more explicit reports about the performance of faculty members involved in their phases and units.

2. Integration of Discipline Concepts Throughout the M.D. Program

While discipline representatives and planners are working together to integrate important concepts into the biomedical problems used in Phases I, II and III, there is need for closer working relationships amongst these groups. Self-evaluation packages need to be prepared for the biomedical problems. The progress being made depends largely upon the interest of the discipline representatives. In Phase V there are plans to alter the purpose of the tutorial so that more emphasis will be placed upon important discipline concepts.

3. Clinical Teaching

The ingredients of clinical teaching have been defined and accepted by the Phase IV Committee. The task will now be one of educating faculty members by workshops and other means, such as direct observation in clinical teaching units. This is an area that we are only beginning to explore.

In addition, I would identify five other changes needed:

i) Students need more unscheduled time to learn on their own.

ii) There is need to resist pressure from groups who want to add fact-filled subjects to the curriculum, unrelated to the biomedical problems.

iii) There is need for better integration of clinical medicine in the early phases, and the basic medical sciences in the clinical phase.

iv) There is need for more behavioral issues to be included in biomedical problems.

v) While a variety of learning resources exist for students, there is need for better linkage with the biomedical problems.

vi) There is a need for a better emphasis on those factors which influence the health of the general population.

What is our Capacity for Change?

From my vantage point our capacity for change is substantial. To date the current resource restraints have not seriously affected the M.D. Program. I would attribute our capacity for change to two factors: people and systems.

1. People

   i)   The support provided by faculty leaders is outstanding. This includes the deanery, departmental chairmen, the Program for Educational Development, and program planners.

   ii) Members of departments, physicians in the community and many institutions have responded positively to our many requests for their involvement.

   iii) The stimulation created by the probing minds of our students brings many rewards. The impact of their involvement in the planning and development of the M.D. Program, as well as ongoing feedback, should not be underestimated.

2. Systems

   i)   The creative tension of the matrix system does much to facilitate change. By having education programs separate from departments, it is possible to develop plans unencumbered by departmental demands. At the same time, planners must be responsive to departmental requests and negotiate resource requirements with departmental chairmen.

   ii) The reward system which requires educational contributions for promotion and tenure has a strong impact upon faculty members.

   iii) The system of the time-limited appointments for leadership roles provides an opportunity for faculty members to become involved in various tasks in the M.D. Program. For example, in the five years since I have been Program Chairman, there has been a new person appointed to every leadership position. Each appointment creates new capacity for change.

iv) A support system exists for faculty members for enhancement of skills in various areas, such as the tutor training workshops and educational courses organized by the Program for Educational Development and the Clinical Epidemiology and Biostatistics course on critical thinking.

v) Finally, the system for regularly reviewing the M.D. Program and its component parts identifies those areas in which changes are needed. Reviews are of two types: internal and external.

Internal. The M.D. Education Committee conducts a review of each part of the M.D. Program every year. In this year (1980) for example, Phase III was reviewed in March and Phase IV will be reviewed in May.

External. External reviews are carried out by both the Health Sciences Education Committee and the Faculty Executive. In the fall of 1980, for example, Faculty Executive established five Task Groups to consider the following important topic areas: evaluation; clinical teaching; academic disciplines; student affairs; and the three-year program. Arising out of the reports were thirty-eight recommendations for the M.D. Program. My earlier comments in this paper on future initiatives was based in large part upon these reports.

Summary

In summary, I have considered change under three headings: changes in the M.D. Program since it began in 1969; changes proposed for the future; and the M.D. Program's capacity for change.

THE DISCUSSIONS: A REVIEW

THE HEALTH SCIENCES NETWORK

by Kerr White, M.D.
Deputy Director, Division of Health Sciences, Rockefeller Foundation
New York, N.Y., U.S.A.

First of all, I want to express my pleasure at having the
opportunity to participate in this 10th Anniversary celebration and to
learn so much from so many colleagues from various parts of the world. I
also want to express my appreciation to Dr. A. Querido and Dr. E. Genton
and also to Dr. J. Cleghorn for the contributions they made to this
summary.

Networks, and particularly health sciences networks, are part of the
current jargon and buzz words which seem to have emerged in the last few
years. It is a felicitous phrase which tends to leave open the usual
questions about authority, control, responsibility, and the traditional
hierarchical and bureaucratic arrangements and regulatory apparatuses
that tend to characterize most human collective enterprises. Although it
is probably premature to attempt to define the concept of the health
sciences network too specifically, there are several characteristics that
seem to have emerged from our discussions. First of all, the network
concept seems to embrace not only aspects of education and services, both
patient services and supporting services, but also aspects of research
and the governance of the entire enterprise. The last three elements
were not discussed as fully as they might have been. The network seems
to consist of a series of nodal institutions, hospitals, agencies, and
probably individuals, and these seem to be linked together by a series of
rather formal and informal commitments. The latter are developed by a
process of negotiation, persuasion, compromise and some limited pecuniary
rewards and recognition of status. Hovering over this entire process are
the external threats of legislative or imposed pressures or sanctions of
one kind or another. It all reminds me a little bit of Rene Dubos'
definition of health which I have found to be the most realistic and
comforting so far: "It is a modus vivendi that permits imperfect

individuals to have a somewhat rewarding and not too painful existence in an imperfect world." The questions at issue during our discussions revolved around the extent to which health sciences networks are flourishing, developing and meeting the needs of the populations they serve, and the extent to which they are likely to grow in influence and effectiveness and be emulated in other areas.

There really are no "solutions" or "answers" to the general agenda we were addressing, there are just experiences to report. Indeed the participants of the health sciences network at McMaster as well as those evolving elsewhere seem to use the network concept to describe an expanding set of nodes and the strengthening of links, but there is also some evidence of fraying ends, of broken strands, and even of shrinking nodes. There are, however, a number of concrete problems and issues that should be addressed and seem to emerge from several different settings. For example, does the university health sciences centre when parachuted into a new community have a different set of problems from the traditional entrenched university that seeks to initiate change both within itself, among its related institutions in the community, and even within those institutions to which it relates? From McMaster, the climate within and among the hospitals and the professions seems to have been particularly opportune for accepting and cooperating, for the most part, with the development of the network, but the same cannot be said for all the other emerging networks in other countries and settings, and it is particularly difficult for the traditional universities to change as dramatically or as rapidly as McMaster. In fact, many of the problems seem almost critical, perhaps severe, but probably not intractable; nevertheless, they remain problems, and you may recall John Updike's aphorism that "problems that have solutions are not problems". There are likely to be continuing problems of one kind or another in virtually every setting, and McMaster will be no exception. Although the problems of a new school or university undertaking the development of a health sciences network may be somewhat easier than those facing an established school, it is bound to have to deal with most of the generic principles, problems and issues that emerged from our discussion.

First of all there is the conceptual issue. Is the university capable of involving itself in all four dimensions of the health care enterprise: education, service, research, and governance? Do all the participants and all of the institutions have the same set of priorities? They may all have the same priorities and objectives but not necessarily the same order of priorities. Is the hidden agenda of the health sciences network really the development of a system of care, a system that is rational with respect to the recognition that there are common problems and rare problems and that there are such relatively identifiable elements as tertiary, secondary and primary care? Is there agreement that there are single networks of care (as well as education, research and governance) that can serve an entire geographic region, and that there can also be competing networks within the same geographic region? This is a difficult notion to understand, but, just as you have Canadian Pacific Airlines and Air Canada fighting for the same markets, so you could have competitive systems operating within the same geographic or catchment area. Do all participants in the network also share the view that there should be some kind of national distribution of the three levels of education – that there should be training for undergraduates, for specialists, and for sub-specialists? The same may be asked of research: Are there places for applied research, for basic research and for health services research?

Second, there are the operational problems. Can the tertiary care of the sub-specialties be divided among the different institutions? Exactly how are they going to be apportioned, as they have with the Hamilton-Wentworth areas where certain hospitals specialize in one function and other hospitals specialize in another subspecialty? Can this be done without substantive implications for practitioners, teachers and administrators, the size of the hospital, the hospital's self-image, for the mixture of their bed complements, for their supporting services?

Matters such as these involve extremely tricky negotiations at all levels of involvement.

Third, there are the implicit or explicit referral patterns within the network. Referring physicians have patterns of long standing and they are not likely to change these readily. There are ticklish problems of admitting, and staff privileges, and appointments at hospitals.

Fourth, there is the question of whether a research agenda with its priorities and funding can be devised and administratively supported so that it will maximize the intellectual capacities and the contributions of all those participating in the network. Will at least some of the research work be on clinical and institutional practices and will it provide guidance for resource allocation to improve the services that are provided? Can investigators at all levels make realistic contributions to the entire network enterprise?

Of course, the final questions that emerge from all this and the ones that cause a good deal of the pain and anxiety are: Who pays for it? By what means are the funds to be channelled? What sums are to be allocated from the different functions? How can all this be accomplished when the institutions and the practitioners seem to have the mission and the responsibility, on the one hand, and the Health Councils — in the case of Ontario — seem to have the authority, and to some extent the political clout, for planning and devising the institutional and service arrangements, but the funds actually flow from provincial sources? These are some of the problems that emerged from the local scene; they seem to be reflected in the experiences of others also.

Let me now discuss in somewhat greater detail these ubiquitous human and institutional conflicts that emerge in most health care settings. There are four necessary, it seems to me, but not necessarily mutually exclusive, means that can be used to varying degrees in different settings to accomplish change. In fact, probably all are required in most settings to establish a health sciences network.

First there is the question of <u>legislation</u>. It may even be asked whether any health sciences network can really be established without a legislative base. There is enabling legislation, regulatory legislation, and managerial legislation; they have all been used in various settings. But without some form of legislation that sooner or later reflects the public's expectations, one questions whether, in fact, an effective network can really be established. As Rudolf Virchow pointed out many years ago, medicine is essentially a social science and politics is nothing but medicine on a grand scale. A corollary to all this is that the governance of the networks and their components sooner or later must reflect the public will and the legislative requirements, or one or the other will be changed. The legislation will be changed, the membership of the network's governing body will be changed, or its charter and its articles of governance will be modified.

That bring us to the second way of effecting change: <u>naked political clout</u>. Attempts to impose the will of the university on the community are not likely to meet with universal acceptance, nor are attempts to impose the will of the community's practitioners on the population served likely to be an unqualified success. The traditions of an outmoded or unbalanced hospital service cannot be continued endlessly. The public is paying for these services, and attempts to invoke past achievements or even the current glories of particular aspects of biomedical, behavioral, or even health services research are not likely to result in uncritical financial or political support if an unbalanced system persists in the educational, research or service dimensions.

There was not as much reference to the third means of effecting change, that is <u>information</u>, as I had anticipated there might be. Indeed it is difficult for me to understand how planning, resource allocation and evaluation can really be carried out without information at the small area level, at the institutional level, and at the regional level, as well as at the provincial and national levels. It seems an essential ingredient for helping to both clarify the issues and identify the difference between cerebral and thalamic responses to any proposals for change advanced from any quarter.

Finally, there is the question of the flow of funds, the control of budgets and the manner in which the money is to be passed from one hand to another. For better or for worse, at least in most western industrialized societies, the power of the purse is still an element to be reckoned with by all concerned.

Without the use of one or more of these four elements - legislation, information, naked political clout, or control of funds - it is difficult to see how much change can be brought about. But whatever is done with respect to all this, there remains the factor of negotiation and compromise and the best ways in which to engage in that process.

Now let me reflect on the four or five major conclusions that emerged from the discussion.

1.   The relationship and motivation to achieve agreement of substance between hospitals and universities is greatly facilitated at the outset if there are identifiable positive forces which encourage both constituencies to enter into the partnership. It would be unfortunate if the emphasis were solely on negative external pressures.

2.   It is probably important to have an affiliation agreement which articulates (although it may be fairly general, initially) the noncontentious elements. One may be able to carry it on to quite comprehensive and detailed documents. And when possible, of course, it is important to develop a document at an early stage so that the successor can understand quite realistically the conditions of the partnership.

At the outset, the focus of activities often succeeds best if it is built around a program of one kind, such as psychiatric services, support services, a burn unit, a renal dialysis or renal transplant unit, open heart surgery, and so forth, rather than around complete institutions, so there can be networks within networks.

97

3.   The plans for education and research activities need to occur in the affiliated hospitals in such a way that they are developed with the full participation and full understanding of the medical staffs. Without this clear understanding, it is almost too much to expect success. It may be best to start with the so-called "teaching unit" initially, but sooner or later the others have to be involved, and it is important that the perception of the arrangements involve full disclosure not only to the medical staff but eventually to the Board and the senior administrators. It is well to recall that recommendations for change in any setting, and certainly within a hospital, are predictably threatening and provoke numerous reactions of resistance. Not all opposition or resistance to change should be interpreted as retarding progress, however, since not all change is necessarily associated with progress. The discussion was given a thumbnail sketch of Machiavelli's contributions to these kinds of deliberations over the years. The relationships between authority and leadership are complicated, but perceptions about the two are very much concerned with actions and interactions or lack of action in other people's behaviour.

4.   There are significant behavioural aspects to all the preceding considerations. From this emerged some basic management principles which, by the use of lateral thinking, could well be embraced in the health care enterprise. For example, there is the use of such basic management principles as identifying and realizing what the problems are and setting mutually understood objectives and solutions. There is also the need to establish trust by open access to information and follow-through on agreements that have been made. Provision of sufficient information so that the rationale for changes or choices is always comprehensible to all of those who are involved, is an essential ingredient. Steps which ensure that the rewards are perceptible and tangible, at least to the extent that there is relief from the discomfort generated by the old system, make change more acceptable.

5. It is important to give careful attention to the timing of proposed changes. The rate of change observed in psychotherapy was referred to and is a helpful guide. Working repetitively at all levels of the system is required. Encouraging participation and decision-making to some degree by all concerned is constructive. This does not necessarily involve participation in studying all the fundamental objectives of the enterprise – that is largely a task of leadership – but it certainly involves giving almost everyone involved opportunities to comment, to reach and to modify and even to propose alternative solutions and perhaps even to dissent. The need for understanding group relationships, the boundaries between groups, and the projection of these perceptions onto the attitudes of the groups, and of events as they occur is important to recognize. It is also important to appreciate that goodwill and altruism are more likely to be effective in new developments than in an old system where entrenchment and vested interest manifest little goodwill; therefore, in the older systems it is essential to find out, nourish and support whatever goodwill exists for contemplated change even more than it is a requirement in new settings.

6. It is important to recognize that the people and their government always have the option of saying "Develop a coordinated system or you will get no money". This is always an unfortunate choice, but the participants may simply have to be told that they must develop some kind of coordinating mechanism if the funds are to flow. Having embarked on this course the community is apt to go from enabling legislation to managerial legislation and eventually to a set of entrenched guidelines that discourage flexibility and innovation. When communication does not solve the problem and simply highlights the differences, then limits of some kind have to be set. Again, political clout is apt to be exercised and more stringent legislation is apt to be enacted. In the last analysis, mustering of public support is good policy; it usually helps professionals to stop their bickering and get on with the job.

The creation of a health sciences network is an evolving exercise. There are no "right" answers; there just seem to be problems and choices. It is a learning experience, for all concerned, and I suppose one can recall Oscar Wilde's aphorism – which might also be an apt description of the McMaster philosophy – that "nothing worth learning can be taught!"

THE DISCUSSIONS: A REVIEW

FACULTY MOTIVATION AND PREPARATION

by Peter F. Regan, M.D.
Professor, Department of Psychiatry and
Director, Health Policy Studies, Faculty of Health Sciences
State University of New York at Buffalo
U.S.A.

Let me add my thanks for the splendid and enjoyable meeting we have
had. The achievements of the McMaster Faculty of Health Sciences have
played a major role in shaping international health care and education
recommendations of the Organizaton for Economic Cooperation and
Development, and the rich exploration of the past days will further
extend McMaster's influence.

At the same time, I must confess that the meeting has had moments of
tension, at least for visiting faculty coordinators. In this morning's
wrap-up session on faculty motivation and preparation, for example, the
planning group piled one paradox on top of another and one complication
on another. Finally, at about a quarter to twelve, Dr. Jack Sibley
exclaimed: "That's the answer! It's creative tension! Everything is
contradictory. Just put it all together and give it!"...and here we are.

What Dr. Sibley said is true. The whole problem of motivation
revolves around a certain paradox and a certain tension. Whenever we
talk about motivation, we are in fact talking about trying to mobilize
the efforts of some individual person to work toward the objectives of
some group or organization. In order to do that we must satisfy that
person. There must be rewarding feedback between an organization and
every individual human person - each one of us, for example. Clearly,
that feedback loop is extremely complicated.

Our discussions over these last three days have added to this
complexity, because we have been looking at a very special case of
motivation. We have dealt with faculty motivation, and more particulary
(on the occasion of this 10th Anniversary) with faculty motivation

101

related to problem-oriented teaching and service networks. That is indeed a special case of motivation. We must recognize it as such so that the satisfaction of other motivational feedback loops can also be maintained.

Apart from problem-oriented teaching and service networks, all faculty members must also have motivation and productivity within their disciplines, within their departments, within their specialties. They also have motivational and feedback loops with family, with neighbourhoods, and with the community. If we jump too far, thinking that motivation for a particular kind of teaching and service network is the answer, we know we are going to fail because we are going to come into conflict with all these other motivational loops. It is in this larger context that our working groups have been dealing with this special case. In order to make the conclusions stand out clearly, I shall start at the human end of the scale to show what motivational forces need to be mobilized, then shift to the organization end to identify what the organization can do about it.

Human Factors in Motivation

Let us begin with the human side of faculty motivation. Our first set of findings on this special case of motivating faculty for problem-oriented teaching and service networks is that these areas are distinguished by a vast lack of support in the ordinary things one thinks of as motivating factors. We heard a little bit of that in Professor David Maddison's address. These kinds of teaching and service networks are not the cherished apple of the academic eye. They are not apt to be enthusiastically rewarded in the universities of the world, so the motivation of academic rank is constrained. Money, as we heard in our first session Monday afternoon, is a motivational force which is virtually missing in the academic world; to the extent that financial rewards are available, they are frequently directed at more traditional achievements. Advancement by mobility is also limited in academic systems that are narrow and closed. It is extremely difficult, for example, to move in the Netherlands where other faculties of the university and government may interpose their wishes on the individual, the group, and the department in medical faculties. It is difficult for francophone colleagues in Quebec to move because of the very limited number of facilities in which they may work. Finally, old institutions with older faculty members can inhibit progress by virtue of tenure and adherence to outmoded ideas.

It is quite apparent, however, that a very significant number of motivational elements are available, and can be valuable if the administrations of health science faculties use them wisely. Albeit one thinks of money as a major motivator to begin with, my friends in social psychology and in management emphasize that real motivation depends on things other than rank and money. This is what our working groups found: keys to motivation that re-emphasized many of the points Professor Maddison made. The promising and successful techniques that we reviewed and analyzed make a substantial list. Let me touch upon them briefly, with some concrete examples:

1.   A reasonable "fit" between a faculty member's aspirations and organizational expectations is the starting point of faculty motivation. If an organization expects a faculty member to spend 80 percent of his time in teaching and the individual expects that he is going to be spending 80 percent of his time in research, there is a bad motivational problem from the start. Proper recruitment, therefore, must seek out individuals with qualifications and needs best suited to institutional needs.

2.   The selection of students is a very powerful part of a motivational feedback loop. Those of you who talked with students here at McMaster will recognize that the students were identifying faculty who could lead and faculty who couldn't lead, and were very verbal and vociferous in their expressions of positive and negative feedback to faculty. At Maastricht, where many other motivational elements are missing, one of

the most moving forces towards change is the quality and the vigor of the students who are continually prodding faculty.

3. A third factor in building motivation lies in making major investments in preparing faculty to do the things that the institution wishes them to do. This preparation requires money, time and space. We have seen the program here at McMaster; it involves worskhops, tutorial preparation and the like. Similar workshops are given at Cali in Colombia, and at New South Wales in Australia. Maastricht finds that it is easier to prepare Netherlands faculty to work in a network by sending them over to Hamilton where they experience it in a foreign situation.

4. A fourth factor is the provision of constant strong technical support. One cannot go up to the Health Sciences Library and to the Learning Resources Centre at McMaster without seeing tangible evidence of the support provided for faculty pursuing the kinds of educational programs that this organization wants. There are excellent physical resources and a library and learning resources staff not only willing but eagerly moving out to help the faculty in innovative activities.

5. Finally, there needs to be a reliable system of human personal recognition for excellence and achievement. This recognition must come at appropriate times and in appropriate places. If you are operating a network as at Cali, for example, you may have to make sure that senior faculty rotate through all nodes of the network, so that workers on one node don't think of themselves as cut off, but as part of a network where there is a feedback loop. If you are redirecting faculty effort to new charges and new duties, there must be some regular reliable review of what they are doing and how well they are doing it. There must be personal interactions with other responsible members of the faculty and students to give them the feedback. Such contact and acknowledgement of merit can be further bolstered by the use of whatever financial or prestige rewards are available. At Maastricht, faculty can be given small bonuses; at other universities they may be given small merit increases in salary; at Trömso, effective faculty members are invited to

join national advisory bodies, and can achieve national prominence in a much more rapid way than if they were at Oslo; at many universities, national and international travel are part of the reward system.

Underlying most of these specific methods for motivating is one phenomenon which deserves special attention: collegiality. Peer reviews, reviews from superiors and students, confidence in support systems, and security in the justice and equity of the reward system depend upon true collegiality. This is not just "good fellowship" and sharing a drink at five o'clock. Instead, it involves a sense of being a vital part of an organization, with the capacity to participate appropriately in the decision-making processes of that organization. Clearly, collegial participation develops the sense of commitment to institutional goals and can help to modify these institutional goals. Collegial participation can also protect people from the fear of change. If faculty are certain that organizational changes will be undertaken only after full discussion and after the facts are on the table, and that tolerances for individuals will be built into the change, there will be much less digging-in of heels that we see so often in institutions that make non-collegial, arbitrary changes.

Organizational Factors in Motivation

Let us now shift from considering elements that motivate faculty members, and view the organizational side of motivation. The working groups felt that a certain number of organizational steps were particularly clear and necessary if all these very varied but incremental motivating elements were to be pulled together. A trip is a good thing for one fellow, a pat on the back is a good thing for another fellow, an opportunity to work on Sunday night is a good thing for another fellow. They are all different.....how does an organization pull them together into a motivational whole?

The working groups recognized a number of ways in which organizations could promote the coherent use of motivational elements.

These techniques are used by a number of participating schools, but
McMaster is outstanding in the degree to which it has adopted the full
range of measures:

1. A major first step is the existence of clearly stated institutional
goals. It is only with a set of well-recognized goals that an
institution can pursue consistent policies with reference to faculty
motivation and reward, as well as with reference to other parts of the
service network, and to the education and health care systems in their
totality.

2. The organizational leaders must ensure faculty participation in
shaping and reshaping institutional goals. As Professor Knut Westlund
emphasized, the most critical role of the dean is to chair and lead those
decisive faculty meetings that map out the future.

3. There must be effective organizational means for involving the
maximum number of faculty and students in administration - the day-to-day
decisions and actions involved in the implementation of goals.

4. It is important to avoid excessive or imbalanced enthusiasm that may
create a feverish amount of motivation for a short period and the
eventual destruction of motivation. One of the major functions of an
administration must be to preserve a balanced array of motivational
forces. Motivation for problem-oriented education and health networks
cannot succeed by sacrificing motivation for contributions to
disciplines, departments and services. Balance must be maintained.

As the working groups reviewed these organizational approaches to
motivation, the issue of institutional age emerged. Is it easier to
create innovation and motivation in an old school or a new one? Those
who come from old institutions say it is much easier in a new
institution, but those in new institutions cite the difficulties of
getting started, fighting the "establishment", etc. In fact, the issues
of motivation are the same in schools new and old. The processes of
change and growth and the processes of maintaining excellence demand the
mobilization of faculty effort. In both new and old institutions there

is an array of motivational elements at hand, as we have seen. The
intelligent dean leading an established school can look at the history of
McMaster and see how a collegial atmosphere can be created, how
organizational steps like the formation of the Program for Educational
Development can begin to cut across disciplinary lines, and how multiple
feedback loops can contribute to solid and dedicated motivation.

Conclusion

The outcome of our deliberations on faculty motivation, therefore,
is an optimistic one. Health science faculties young and old, as they
enter the 1980's, have at hand an array of effective motivational tools.
The secret of success is using those tools coherently and cohesively, and
McMaster University's Faculty of Health Sciences stands out as a model of
how this can be done.

THE DISCUSSIONS: A REVIEW

RESEARCH IN THE HEALTH SCIENCES NETWORK

by Stephen Leeder, M.D.
Professor of Community Medicine
University of Newcastle
New South Wales, Australia

The discussions in the last three days with respect to the role of research in the health sciences network have been characterized by a high degree of enthusiasm and much flexibility. A multiplicity of viewpoints were expressed by representatives from different cultural backgrounds including Canada, the United States, Nigeria, Thailand, several European countries, and Australia. The discussion was wide-ranging, but all the viewpoints had a practical focus.

I wish to present the findings and considerations of the groups which looked at research as answers to five questions:

1. What is meant by research?

2. What is the role of a network university with regard to research?

3. What are the factors and biases influencing the choice of research problems and priorities?

4. Who should do research?

5. How should research be organized?

What is Meant by Research?

Perhaps it is easy to begin by saying what we do not mean by research. We do not construe "research" to be synonymous with "science." It is, instead, a much more operational term which applies to the flexible implementation of science for a variety of goals which may include education, service and the advancement of knowledge. While there is much debate about the way science should be made operational through research, there was, in the group, no debate about the fundamental ethical aspects of science.

We accepted the view put forward by Medawar that there are many
forms of science and indeed many more forms of research. We agreed that
no one form of science should be seen as exclusive of others, or
considered sufficient for the conduct of all forms of research. There
was a general plea to avoid a reductionist view of science. Science
could on occasion be carried out through "thought experiments," as it was
by Einstein, without any research at all. On the other hand, health
services research requires the development of an appropriate methodology
for problem-solving rather than the development of highly imaginative
research questions.

What is the Role of a Network University with Regard to Research?

Several roles were defined. The university, as a tertiary
institution and bastion of preservation of critical thinking, has science
as one of its key attributes, and its role must be that of guardian of
scientific purity. While research can be carried out by non-academic
institutes and statutory health departments, the contribution of a
university is to maintain high levels of science in the research with
which it is associated.

There is also an important educational role for the network
university in the development of critical approaches in all members of
the network associated with the university.

Another fundamental role of a network university is the application
of research to service, as we heard in descriptions of its usefulness in
understanding Nigerian health problems, its use in the Regional Service
Program at McMaster, and indeed its usefulness in ecological research
among Karen hill tribes in Thailand. An interesting reciprocity existed
here between the research and the object being researched — not only was
knowledge being advanced by the research, but important implications for
manpower planning were perceived as a result of the new insights and
definitions of health problems which then influenced the educational
programs being offered for health professionals.

What are the Factors and Biases Influencing the Choice of Research Problems?

These factors and biases can be divided into three groups. The first is ideology. After World War II, there was heavy emphasis upon explanatory science, where the orginality of the idea rather than the methodology for testing it was rewarded. There was de-emphasis upon predictive or prognostic research, of which epidemiological forms of enquiry are examples. Now, however, an ideological shift is occurring, and increasing emphasis is being placed upon epidemiological and qaulitative research into, for example, quality of life and the quality of health care provided. This shift to population-based research makes the network as important to the researcher as the researcher is to the network, for without well-informed critical data gatherers, such research cannot succeed. This kind of research places a major emphasis on the development of methodological strategies and ways in which outcomes can be measured, and it is here, rather than in the development of a creative or complicated question, that most energy is invested.

Ideological factors can operate internationally, nationally or locally to influence the choice of research problems and the priorities assigned to them.

The second major factor influencing the choice of research priorities was seen to be money. Some participants complained that the balkanisation of research monies occurring in some countries which lack national health research policies was leading to a loss of research coherence. Others complained that the current three-year funding system for project grants "ground down" creativity, as though all research projects could be neatly fitted into a three-year period. It was generally accepted that political lobbying is necessary to change these situations.

The third major factor influencing choice of problems is charisma! A powerful departmental head, by virtue of salesmanship, can determine research priorities and focus on problems which are then considered worthy of support.

Who Should do Research?

Research is an activity which should be shared. Medical students should do it - and here we see an important example of the way in which research can be used for educational goals rather than the advancement of knowledge as a primary goal. At Southampton 70 percent of one year of the course is devoted to a research project; similarly, students in Nigeria carry out "hands on" research. It was debated whether it was necessary for students to experience the emotional consequences of attempting to carry out research or whether they could learn enough about science from watching others do it or simply writing research protocols.

There was general agreement that other members of the network should be involved in research as a learning experience, whether these be other doctors working in associated hospitals (as at McMaster), other health professionals, or non-professionals and consultees as in the Regional Service Program at McMaster.

The importance of maintaining the research and scientific flame through appropriate programs of graduate and post-graduate research was also emphasized.

How Should Research be Organized?

Some questioned whether research should be organized at all, whether organization would limit the creativity of research. Certainly there was agreement that if the Faculty places a high priority on collaborative and programmatic research, which may well make sense on analysis of contemporary health needs and problems facing the network, then recruitment and reward need to favour those managerial structures required for such research.

There was no question that wherever possible, education, research and service should be integrated. Grand Rounds might be used as an outcome evaluation of the extent to which researchers truly integrate their critical research thinking into clinical practice.

Summary

1. Research is the term given to those human activities by which science is operationalized in attempts to solve problems. It comprises a wide range of activities which are, however, limited by the common ethical constraints of science, and have many shared features.

2. Research is vital to the community for many reasons, not only to solve immediate problems but to develop attitudes and critical approaches.

3. Research is affected by various biases which tend to influence the choice of research problems and priority. Some of these are amenable to change; others simply require recognition and avoidance.

4. Research is seen to be not an exlusive activity of a selected priesthood but rather something that should be engaged in to varying extents by many people. The role of "gurus" was nevertheless important, and not to be belittled.

5. Research should be organized loosely, but be in line with Faculty and major network goals.

Science is the stuff of rational innovation. It is very hard to see how progress can occur in a network or in the development of relevant medical educational programs without science as an underpinning methodology, and I for one see no alternative method to research in making our most creative and equitable contribution to communities and our network colleagues within them.

THE DISCUSSIONS: A REVIEW

EDUCATION IN THE HEALTH SCIENCES NETWORK

by Steven Jonas, M.D.
Associate Professor, Department of Community and Preventive Medicine
School of Medicine, State University of New York at Stony Brook
Long Island, New York, U.S.A.

I found this a most exciting conference, being able to meet many
people from all around the world who are active in changing medical
education. I will present some of the problems and questions that have
been raised in the discussions of the medical education program at
McMaster in two sets. The first set will be matters for which fairly
clear answers and/or solutions appear to exist; the second set will be
matters for which answers and/or solutions are still to be developed
and/or the problem has not yet been addressed. The problems on the list
have arisen out of the McMaster experience, but for the most part they
and their solution can be generalized to the world experience.

Clearly-Defined Issues

1. Student Anxiety

First of all we consider the problem of the anxiety level of medical
students at McMaster, i.e. the anxiety level of medical students working
in a problem-based learning curriculum. In commenting, one can say that
medical school is an anxiety-provoking experience no matter how you do
it. At McMaster there seems to be a constant source of stress in not
knowing precisely where you stand. At conventional schools, however, the
stress is precisely in knowing where you stand and in going through the
frequent exercises designed to tell you that. Further, at McMaster the
students' anxiety is internally generated. At conventional schools it is
externally generated.

2. Gaps in Learning

The second problem concerns supposed learning gaps in knowledge and lack of opportunities or requirement for study in depth, particularly in the basic sciences. In response, it can be noted that all medical students and all doctors have gaps in their knowledge and in their competencies. Any student who goes to a conventional medical school, which does not have written learning objectives and grades its students on the normal distribution curve in which 65 is a passing grade, has gaps – even if the student's memory for what he or she memorizes for the exam is indefinite (which in most cases it isn't). At least the McMaster students are taught how to fill the gaps at the time they need to be filled, and there are, in fact, opportunities made available for exploration in depth which are related to learning objectives. Furthermore, what is taught in the whole curriculum is based on learning objectives which in turn are derived from the needs of clinical practice, not from the customary academic mode of "What do I know, therefore what do I teach?" Another description of the conventional approach to teaching in medical education is a paraphrase I have developed of Dr. Kerr White's description of clinical practice in an era of specialization. Dr. White described a clinical encounter as the patient saying "I hope he treats what I've got" and the specialist saying "I hope he's got what I treat." The parallel in conventional medical schools is the student saying "I hope he teaches what I need" and the teacher saying "I hope he needs what I teach."

3. The Three-Year Curriculum

The third identified problem is the three-year lock-step curriculum and its apparent lack of flexibility. However, because of the problem-based learning system there is at least flexibility within the various phases. Furthermore, elective time is relatively generous and not just saved up for the end, as it is in most medical schools where it often simply enhances the drive to early specialization. Special problems of students who evidently need more than the two years and nine months to finish the program are, in fact, dealt with on a case-by-case basis.

4. Interprofessional Education

Next, the problems and successes of interprofessional education are discussed. The experience has been that most success in this endeavour has occurred when the objectives of the interprofessional education are content-oriented, e.g. when doctors and nurses are studying together history-taking and physical examination. When the objectives deal with role definition in the health care personnel hierarchy, the exercises are not so successful.

5. Problem-Solving in the Clerkship

The fifth problem identified arises out of the introduction of problem-based learning into Phase IV, the Clinical Clerkships. We were told that McMaster is making a determined effort to deal with this problem. I should tell you that when I made my first visit to McMaster in 1974 and was immersed in problem-based learning, I attended a very stimulating Phase I tutorial at the home of one of the faculty members. There was another tutor present at that session. After the tutorial was over, I told them both how excited I was by the experience and went on to ask, "Well, what do you think the problems are?" One of the faculty members answered "Well, our most serious problem (and this was in 1974) is how to introduce problem-based learning into Phase IV, and by God, we are going to deal with it!" They are still working on that one.

I think that the solution to the Phase IV problem lies in the aggressive use of the problem-oriented medical record and the problem-oriented approach to the evaluation of quality of clinical performance. This requires doctors and students to continually justify their approaches to data base gathering, the problem set, clinical reasoning, the investigations proposed, and the interventions proposed, against previously agreed-upon standards of care.

The problem-oriented record, it seems to me, is the natural clinical analogue of the problem-based learning approach and allows problem-based learning to continue life-long in the clinical setting. McMaster is re-looking at Phase IV now and will be introducing the "critical appraisal of data" approach in an attempt to make it more rigorous. The critcal appraisal of data approach in teaching in this area is strongly featured in the medical school at Beer-Sheva, Israel.

6. Flexibility

The sixth problem is that of maintaining flexibility in the program. The solutions which seem to exist for that problem lie in not being overly defensive, evaluating criticism carefully, and looking at external experience while at the same time keeping one's eye on the ball.

Less Well-Defined Issues

I will turn now to some of the problems for which answers are not yet so readily apparent.

1. Self-Directed Learning

The "guided discovery" and self-directed learning, in which McMaster prides itself, are, to my view, more guided and structured than faculty here care to admit. I think that structure, particularly related to learning objectives, is a good thing. Learning objectives are set, problems are designed to cover the objectives, and although solution of all problems is not required of all students, most of the students, in fact, do most of the problems. Therefore, in the environment of setting learning objectives and requiring a structured approach to achieving those learning objectives (despite the fact that faculty will tell you how unstructured they are), those learning objectives are expected to be achieved.

2. Basic Orientation: Disease or Health?

The second problem in this group that I see is that the basic disease orientation of the ideological content of western medical education has been so far maintained in the McMaster context. It seems to me that health orientation is the logical next step in the development of medical education.[1] Problem-based learning is indeed essential to it, since when dealing with health promotion and disease prevention in individuals and populations, one is dealing more often than not with problems, not with diagnosis. Beer-Sheva and the medical school at

Newcastle, New South Wales, both are health-oriented. The Texas College of Osteopathic Medicine in Forth Worth is planning to be the first North American School to move in this direction.[2]

3. Outcome Assessment

Next arises the question of "Does it make any difference?" In other words, is it really worthwhile having McMaster go to all this trouble both in its very complex admissions process and also its very complex curriculum? Now there is a division of opinion on this one. Some people think that McMaster has been very remiss in its evaluation efforts and that it should already have at least some answers to this question. Others say that it is too early to make these kind of judgments, that having graduated only six classes — which means that only the members of the first two or three classes (which in fact had very small numbers of people in them) are actually out in clinical practice — makes it too soon to undertake such evaluation.

In fact, McMaster has done some objective evaluation of its program, e.g. reviewing the performance of its students on standardized tests both at the immediate postgraduate and the postspecialty board levels, where they seem to do well in comparison with other graduates of other Canadian schools. Furthermore, there have been attempts to get other medical schools to agree to have their graduates interviewed on a single-blind basis by outside observers against McMaster graduates, and so far, at least, other schools have been unwilling to cooperate in this effort.

4. Emphasis on Health Care Systems

We did not hear that health planning and policy analysis questions related to the training program have been addressed. Important policy issues are, for example, health manpower planning which, as Professor A. Querido pointed out on the first day, is so critical to health care delivery system planning, the forms of medical practice, and the patterns of physician reimbursement. There has been research on the use of nurse practitioners in primary care. In fact, McMaster has the only remaining nurse practitioner program in Canada. However, in the future doctors may

117

be replaced in primary care by the nurse practitioner/physician's associate type of person. Research has increasingly shown this to be a feasible and cost-effective alternative.[3] If this were to happen, then the McMaster type of learning is essential, in my view, for the higher-level role of the doctor in primary care, which would be in supervision, education, research, referral, and evaluation. However, it seems to me that it would be very fruitful for McMaster to formally study some of these questions.

5. The Evaluation Dilemma

Finally in the problem list of unanswered questions is the dilemma of having formative, i.e. "help the student," evaluation and summative, i.e. "decision on passing," evaluation going on simultaneously. This is a question which needs more study.

Concluding Remarks

I have two final comments. First, the change in the medical education process done at McMaster and at Maastricht is necessary because of well-demonstrated deficits in the quality of patient care which are related to how doctors practice medicine. That is, these changes do not arise and are not necessary simply because somebody thinks that they are a good idea or that they fit rationally into educational theory. They arise and they are needed because there is something that is not productive for the health of the people that is related to the educational process, and therefore the educational process needs change. Changes as well in the content of medical education, i.e. changing to a health orientation, as at Beer-Sheva and Newcastle, are also made necessary by objective material circumstances, that is, the primacy of prevention in improving the health of the people.

Second, Dr. Harmen Tiddens in his opening talk expressed concern over the slowness of change. In the historical perspective of change in medical education, I think that we are, in fact, moving quite rapidly. McMaster opened ten years ago. In my country, change in medical education seems to be on a one-hundred-year cycle. Focusing around the year 1800, there was a change from preceptor-only medical education to the appearance of medical schools. Preceptor training as a sole source of medical education, in fact, did not disappear in the United States until the late 19th century, and of course we retain its positive features in our present bedside clinical teaching modes. Focusing around the year 1900, there was change from the 19th century type of generally unplanned, unorganized medical education in medical schools to a university-based graded instruction system with laboratories, clinical teaching, and prerequisites for admission, the so-called Flexnerian reforms. It happens that the first report making recommendations which are, in fact, similar to those that appeared in the Flexner report in 1910 was issued in 1827. It was produced by the first meeting of representatives of American medical schools interested in the problems of medical education. The first school of the type which eventually became accepted in this century as conventional, that is the so-called "Flexnerian school" (actually a complete misinterpretation of what Flexner was talking about), was opened in 1858 at Lind University in Chicago, Illinois. That medical school eventually became part of Northwestern University.

The changes that focused around 1900 occurred when they did because of changes in the nature of medical practice related to the growth of scientific knowledge and the oversupply of doctors. Now that is a simplification, but we see that there were real, objective, material requirements at that time for change in medical education relating both to the doctor supply and to the quality of the work that was being done.

If we project that this one-hundred-year cycle will continue, and I think that it probably will, then the next stage of change, which will be to the health-oriented, problem-based learning approach, will occur focusing around the year 2000. Interestingly enough, it will once again be related to real material objective requirements, i.e. changes in scientific knowledge, this time in the epidemiologic understanding of the basis of chronic disease and, in the United States at least, the oversupply of doctors. If we say that we are expecting to see changes focusing around the year 2000 and we argue by historical analogy, then considering that the first prototype school for the 21st century began its program in 1970, I think we are on the right track.

References

[1]Jonas, S. Medical Mystery: The Training of Doctors in the United States. New York: W.W. Norton, 1979.

[2]Texas College of Osteopathic Medicine. Design of the Medical Curriculum in Relation to the Health Needs of the Nation. Fort Worth, Tx., 1980.

[3]Record, J.C. et al. The New Health Practitioner in Primary Care: Provider Requirements and Cost Savings. New York: Springer Publishing Co., 1981 in press.

THE DISCUSSIONS: A REVIEW

SUMMARY OF DISCUSSIONS

by John Evans, M.D.
Director, Department of Population, Health and Nutrition,
International Bank for Reconstruction and Development
Washington, D.C., U.S.A.
Dr. Evans was founding dean of McMaster's School of Medicine

Dean Mustard, Ladies and Gentlemen. It is a very special privilege not only to rejoin my colleagues at McMaster but also to meet with those engaged in the development of new health sciences programs elsewhere and to share their experiences and impressions which relate so closely to those which marked the early years of the McMaster program. What strikes me most forcefully is the similarity in motivation for your educational innovations: unmet health needs in your own communities and the importance of reshaping eductional programs to meet those needs. It was not an attempt to find a specific new model of medical education since it in turn would soon become as obsolete as the programs you are attempting to replace.

It is a great pleasure to see one person here who showed exceptional courage in encouraging the group in the health sciences to undertake the McMaster experiment. Dr. Harry Thode, president of McMaster University when this experiment was started, had to cope with community reaction, closure of Hamilton's main thoroughfare, dismissal of conventional experienced architects, and a host of practical problems caused by an inexperienced group of enthusiasts. At the same time, we had to steer through the University senate an unconventional, indeed incomprehensible, curriculum, and appointments for staff without the usual academic credentials. Dr. Thode did this in health sciences as he had done in other divisions of the University with his keen personal interest and support. In looking back on the McMaster experience, one must marvel at the tolerance of the University, the tolerance of the community, and even the tolerance of the Government. I suspect that in each of the situations in which you find yourselves, the same problems exist, but you may not have enjoyed the good fortune to have the same tolerance that we experienced here.

Your discussions have been summarized by the reporters' group. I have been asked to do a summary of a summary. I will use that as part of the base of information but I would also like to use two other sources. A very short questionnaire has been given to representatives from 25 centres here to ask them to identify the outstanding problems and opportunities in the 1980's for their institutions. I will comment on the key issues identified by them. Finally, I will refer to some of the problems which confront me in assisting the World Bank to launch its program of assistance to develop population, health and nutrition in the developing world.

The responses to the questionnaire on problems and opportunities in the 1980's showed much common ground. The most common problem identified by 11 of the 25 visitors was faculty motivation: rewards, training for their role, bucking traditional thinking, the problem of maintaining the momentum and, as one observer put it, faculty fatigue. This issue has been the focus of Dr. Peter Regan's remarks. The second problem, identified by 6 of the group of 25, was funding constraints and the related issues, such as the inability to retain physicians in public sector jobs.

Of the opportunities, there were two recognized by approximately one-third of the respondents. The first was the opportunity to participate in the development of an exemplary health system. I presume "system" was used in the sense explained by Dr. Kerr White as a balanced network of health services to meet the total health needs of a population. The second was the opportunity for educational innovation because of dissatisfaction with current practices.

Phases in the Evolution of Health Services

It is not easy, after the event, to find a theme for my remarks that fits with what has transpired during this conference. Looking at the different situations around the world, one might conclude that there have been phases in the evolution of health services which relate closely to the stages of development of countries. These phases reflect the chief causes of mortality and morbidity during these periods.

In developed countries during the latter part of the last century, communicable diseases and malnutrition were the principal problems. They were manifested by acute illness and overcome primarily by improvement in living standards and income and the introduction of immunization and vector control.

In developed countries we are now in the second phase, which I will label the phase of physical/chemical pathology; cancer, cardiovascular disease, high blood pressure, diabetes, and motor accidents have replaced the elements of the first phase as the principal causes of morbidity and mortality. We have mobilized technological interventions, drugs, and surgery and have spent enormous resources in trying to cope with these diseases. There is some evidence that the second phase is now beginning to recede in terms of stroke and heart disease, but we may be just at the beginning of that recession.

We may be entering the third phase which might be described as the phase of social pathology, using social pathology in its very broadest role: the diseases of human behavior, self-inflicted abuse, violence, suicide, drugs, alcohol, smoking, environmental hazards, the problems of the aged, absenteeism and the problems of the work place which have emerged as prime health and social issues in many countries of Europe and America. Holland represents an interesting example of the entry into this third phase of health in relation to social development. Holland spends more than a thousand dollars per capita on health. There are health services available within five to ten minutes for anybody in Holland. By the conventional indices it has the third best infant mortality rate, second best perinatal mortality rate and lowest maternal mortality rate in the world. It has an average life expectancy of over 74 years, combined for males and females. Its ranking by conventional health indices is very high. But 20 percent of its work force is away from the work place at any given time; half of the 20 percent is on disability insurance and half on sickness insurance.

Dr. Mahler, director general of the World Health Organization (WHO), points out that one-third of adult Danes wake up on tranquilizers each morning, that one-third of Swedish adolescents wake up with alcoholic hangovers, and I can point out that one-third of Canadians don't wake up at all in the morning! The problem of teenage pregnancy is now giving way to pre-teen pregnancy. These observations indicate serious social problems, social pathology, that go beyond the conventional physical/chemical pathology that we are accustomed to deal with. It has been suggested that the relationship between health and development is bimodal; that in the early stages, with improvement of income and living standards, there is a significant improvement in health, but beyond a certain level of income the effect on health is negative. It seems that deterioration in health status with further development is a disability of disposable income.

The question of whether we are using the right indicators for health is illustrated by the example of Holland. They were certainly useful for the first phase and the second phase of evolution, but are they appropriate for the third phase? We are poorly prepared to deal with this third phase in our educational programs, in our clinical teaching units, and in the role models that we have as leaders in our educational problems. So far, only a meager proportion of our research effort is addressed to the problems of this third phase. We do not have in most of our health centers the skills required to begin to look at these problems. Finally, only a minor fraction of our total health resources are spent on dealing with the problems of this third phase, compared to what we have committed to the secondary and tertiary health services of the second phase.

Developed countries seem to be moving from the second phase into the third phase. But developing countries have to deal with all three phases simultaneously: Phase I in rural areas and in peri-urban slums; Phase II in the influential urban middle class; and Phase III in populations with recent increases in disposable income. If it is difficult to cope with Phase III, what a challenge it is to try to cope with all three phases simultaneously!

Population-Based Perspective of Health Care

We have a system which really is still strongly oriented to diseases and to the individual. It seems so much more difficult to think and act in relation to health and to the community, the work place, the family, the environmental aspects of health and disease. The reports at this meeting indicated interesting and encouraging directions underway in Beer-Sheva, Israel and New South Wales, Australia in this respect.

Our system of health care is passive; it waits for the individual to seek help. We must work towards a population-based approach for our health services and health promotion. First, we should assess the nature of the burden of illness and the total health needs of the entire population of a community. Second, we should assess the total resources available and how effectively they are being used to address these needs. Fundamental to this process is a simple information base, available at the level where decisions are taken, which tells us more about the prevalence of disease, which may identify extrinsic factors causing disease, which tells us more about the effectiveness of interventions, including compliance in treatment. These elements are missing from our health services and from the clinical environment in which we train our students. We tend to think that a large percentage of care in our communities is delivered by the medical profession. In developing countries it has been estimated that 80 percent of health care is delivered through "unofficial" channels: herbalists, traditional healers, drug dispensers, injectionists. Even in developed countries, druggists, chiropractors, influential personalities in a community and friends are frequent sources of medical advice. In Ontario, a survey in the 1960's indicated that appoximately one-third of patients seeking psychiatric care consulted ministers first. The most effective programs of health education in developing countries seem to be carried out by school teachers, not the health professions. If we are to reach the population that is at risk and to address the problem of social pathology, we must harness the talents of all sorts of people who are outside the conventionally defined health team. One effort in this direction at McMaster was the recurrent educational program in Clinical Behavioural Sciences in which ministers, social workers and health personnel trained together to improve their skills in handling the health problems they encountered in their jobs outside the health system.

Total community health needs and the population-based approaches place new demands for techniques of measurement of health and management of human and material resources. These skills are needed to assemble evidence for decision-making, to implement the decisions, to monitor progress and to make necessary mid-course corrections. Does this mean new categories of specialists trained exclusively in these areas? There will certainly be some new specialists in these fields, but the major impact on the delivery of health services will come from inculcating these skills in a large variety of the people who have clinical responsibility and who regularly make decisions about the use of resources in our health system. About 80 percent of the resources devoted to health care are influenced by doctors' decisions, but this is one aspect that does not get managed. It will be difficult to manage by external directions; there is a greater chance of success if those responsible for the decisions have the responsibility to gather the evidence and to apply the resources available to the highest priority needs. It would be unrealistic to expect them to be advocates for reduction in resources, but it would be disappointing if they did not rise to the challenge of marshalling available resources to achieve the optimal health outcome.

In speaking of systems of health care, I am not referring to small pilot projects but to a large population base, preferably an entire political jurisdiction. We have learned a lot from pilot projects, but unfortunately pilot projects exist in a political vacuum, and do not reflect the political, administrative and financial realities of large scale implementation. Medical schools and health sciences groups must work with those realities of the large community if they want to contribute to preventive health measures and more rational, population-based approaches to disease detection and management and resource use. In this respect, the separation of clinical health services and public health is both artificial and undesirable. Clinical health services have the vehicle without the message, and public health has the message without the vehicle. Both are important and the community cannot afford the luxury of lack of cooperation of these two groups. As noted by Dr. Kerr White in 1972, what is needed is individuals who combine "commitment to medicine's clinical and social problems. What distinguishes them from colleagues who work only at the bedside, in the clinic or in the laboratory is their focus on the health problems of populations. They are distinguished also from their colleagues in traditional public health by their concern for all personal health services that impinge on populations."

Motivations of Faculty

Returning to the outstanding problems in the 1980's which you have identified for your institutions, the most important was faculty motivation. The problem in the 1980's is not finding innovative ideas; it is finding people who are prepared to carry out those ideas and maintain their enthusiasm for the task against formidable obstacles. As Dr. Regan and the respondents to the questionnaire pointed out, this is the most difficult problem to solve.

First, the criteria for recruiting faculty may be flawed. Universities place academic excellence ahead of all other considerations, and this aspect of the quality of staff is one of the most important elements in the image of the institution. But many individuals who are academically excellent will not be comfortable with programs in education and health care that give priority to institutional objectives at the expense of their discipline. If recruitment is influenced too strongly by concern for external image, it will distort the objectives of the school. If the objectives are faithfully observed in the recruitment process, some academic stars may be lost. This latter option was followed at McMaster and conferred the advantage that a large majority of the staff began with a familiarity with and commitment to the School's unusual objectives. However, almost every new faculty member suffered a relapse to conventional objectives within six months and for this reason it was necessary to reinforce actively the commitment to objectives on an ongoing basis and to ensure that faculty recognition rewarded service to those objectives.

Dr. Regan has summarized the means available to motivate faculty. They are very limited. For many faculty the most important motivating factors are outside the institution - international scientific recognition, clinical prestige and consulting assignments. It is necessary to balance this influence with rewards and recognition that relate to the institutional objectives and if possible make the two sources of motivations parallel, i.e. international eminence through the pursuit of goals of local relevance.

Two of Dr. Regan's points warrant special emphasis. Collegiality is a powerful motivating factor and is strengthened greatly by broad participation of faculty in shaping institutional objectives and in making important decisions. Secondly, resource allocation must be seen to match with institutional objectives and not be distorted by the power structure of the institution. In traditional organizations, the decisions on resource allocation are taken in respect to disciplines and departments, not to institutional program objectives in education, research and health service. At McMaster we organized a matrix system of

128

management in which the department earned its resources by virtue of its contribution to institutional programs. In the same vein, individual faculty recognition in salary and promotion was based in large measure on the assessment by each program director of the individual's contribution to the institution's programs. Matrix organization may not be the best management system, but one of its strengths is the constant reminder to faculty members that working for institutional objectives brings the rewards.

Motivation of Students

As with faculty, the process of selection may be the most important factor in the motivation of students to the objectives which the institution is attempting to achieve. Once again, disproportinate attention to academic achievement and neglect of attitudes and ability to relate to people may produce a class of students who will be ill at ease or antagonistic to the unconventional objectives.

Once admitted, the students will quickly sense what the priorities really are from the shape of the curriculum and the attitudes of the faculty. It is not effective to tell them that social, behavioral and humanistic aspects of medicine are extremely important when only 4 of 132 core courses deal with these subjects and these subjects find scant expression in the clinical work of faculty instructors and residents. It makes little impression to advocate primary health care, partnership with other health workers and a population-based approach if all their clinical role models practice exclusively in hospitals. In this respect, the attempts to take clinical teaching right into the community at Beer-Sheva, Cali (Colombia) and Ilorin (Nigeria), and the experiment in group medicine at the University of Newcastle (Australia) are extremely important innovations.

Our tendency is to focus all our innovative efforts on the under-graduate period of medical education. But, in developed countries, postgraduate or residency training is far more influential in moulding

129

attitudes and clinical practices. The benefits of efforts made at the undergraduate level are certain to be lost unless comparable objectives and experiences are sustained during residency training. For example, we need apprenticeship experience in the epidemiological evaluation of evidence and the management of human and materials resources as part of the clinical training of most residents to improve their effectiveness in patient management and use of resources.

Community medicine and social pathology are difficult to teach. They can be in the mainstream of medical education or a sideshow. If they are the exclusive responsibility of a department of preventive or social medicine, no matter how well they are done they will be treated as a sideshow. Unless they become an objective of the whole medical school, with responsibility shared among most of the departments – particularly the clinical departments – the subjects will be relegated to secondary consideration by medical students, faculty and administration. When the role model is a neurosurgeon, a King's Scholar in his country, who directs his attention to the health problems of the hill tribes of his country, then students and colleagues place this work in the mainstream of their value system.

If medical schools are going to be the flagship of the health sciences fleet, they are going to have to show more leadership and more willingness to cooperate with the other health sciences. Medical schools now have about 90 percent of the resources, but do not produce 90 percent of the benefits. And flagships have a tendency to become obsolete! A vital element in leadership will be the introduction and evaluation of new concepts and approaches. Medical education cannot remain static. The need to motivate the faculty remains absolutely critical. Change will be achieved step by step by a sustained effort and built on areas of strength, not weakness.

In each of your countries the medical schools or the health science centres have an extremely important role in the evolution of health care, whether in a developing country facing all three phases of the health process simultaneously, or in a developed country in transition from the second to the third phase of evolution. There are few institutions that can provide the type of leadership that is necessary. A heavy burden falls on the "new schools" to sustain the efforts you have initiated and to broaden the impact of any successes to the health system as a whole in your country. We all wish you success in sustaining the commitment and enthusiasm of the students and faculty in your institutions which is so vital to the achievement of your objectives.

APPENDIX A

THE McMASTER M.D. PROGRAM:
DESCRIPTION AND DATA

CONTENTS

BASIC PREMISES OF THE McMASTER M.D. PROGRAM

These premises arose out of the strong beliefs of the early planners at the McMaster Medical School that we should be innovative and prepared to experiment. Dissatisfaction with: traditional course work, consisting largely of lectures and laboratory exercises; admission to medical school chiefly on the basis of high grades in science courses; emphasis on achieving high marks in content-oriented examinations; and a tendency to stress teaching while paying little attention to helping students learn, lay behind much of the early thinking.

Premise # 1

A curriculum which is based on biomedical problems, and stresses acquiring knowledge to solve problems, will help to establish a life-long pattern of questioning, seeking and formulating solutions.

Expressions:
a) The core curriculum consists of a series of biomedical problems.

b) Students learn to: identify major issues and questions in problems; hypothesize; seek information; formulate solutions.

Premise # 2

Interweaving basic science and clinical medicine from the outset helps students learn to approach clinical problems with the methods, general principles, and pertinent facts of basic science.

Expressions:
a) From the outset there is a blend of clinical and basic science.

b) Pertinent clinical situations are used to introduce concepts of basic science.

Premise # 3

Too much teaching may inhibit learning how to learn what one needs to know; students need unscheduled time to learn on their own.

Expressions:
a) No mandatory laboratory sessions.
b) Few lectures.
c) Students schedule own activities.

Premise # 4

Different ways of learning are to be encouraged and require a variety of learning resources.

Expressions: a) Faculty have prepared or provided a wide variety of learning resources: monographs, journals, reprints of articles; slide/tape programs, videotapes, dissections, pathological specimens, charts, models, etc.

b) These are catalogued and stored for quick access.

c) Students are encouraged to approach problems in individual ways. Small group tutorials can facilitate varied approaches to learning.

Premise # 5

In order to cope with increasingly complex problems in the future, society needs doctors with diverse attitudes and backgrounds.

Expressions: a) Students are selected with diverse educational and work backgrounds.

b) Able students need not have a science background at university before admission.

Premise # 6

Students can learn from each other and from tutors who are fellow-learners.

Expressions: a) The class is divided into groups of five with a faculty tutor who is familiar with the topics but not necessarily expert, and wishes to learn more.

b) Attention is paid to the individual styles of students and tutors and to group dynamics in order to promote effective learning in the group.

Premise # 7

Doctors work more and more in groups which include a variety of health professionals. Practice increases effectiveness as a group member.

Expressions: a) In tutorials participants should learn to recognize behaviour which facilitates and stimulates productivity and to avoid behaviour which inhibits progress in the group.

b) Students observe and take part in various groups in community practice, hospital work, medical school planning and research.

Premise # 8

Empathy and compassion can be enhanced by interviewing skills and understanding of behaviour.

Expressions: a) Interviewing skills are learned in small groups with expert preceptors.

b) Behavioural issues are included in biomedical problems.

Premise # 9

A three-year medical course should be sufficient to prepare most students for postgraduate work.

Expressions: a) By limiting summer holidays to one month, 31 months are available compared to the usual 34 months of a four-year course.

b) The same financial assistance is available from government over the three years as is provided for students in four-year courses.

c) Details of such fact-filled subjects as anatomy and biochemistry are reduced by requiring students to learn only what is needed to deal with the biomedical problems.

Premise # 10

Students benefit by opportunities to select experiences for themselves, explore subjects in more depth and try novel approaches.

Epxressions: a) A wide variety of electives are available.

b) Blocks total 26 weeks.

c) These electives enable students to explore areas of interest or, where necessary, do remedial work on topics in which they are deficient.

Premise # 11

Competition for marks, standing, prizes and scholarships inhibits co-operative learning and encourages note memorization and cramming.

Expressions: a) There are no examinations with marks, or class standings, or prizes. Students are identified as satisfactory or unsatisfactory in each unit.

b) Monies for scholarships and bursaries are awarded on the basis of financial need.

Premise # 12

Faculty and students will be more enthusiastic about learning if both have responsibility for planning a flexible curriculum.

Expressions: a) Phase and unit faculty planners and students are chosen to be responsible for segments of the course. Choice is made on the basis of aptitude and interest, without regard to seniority.

b) Departmental chairmen are responsible for deploying their staff throughout the course, but have no official responsibility for content.

c) No courses are provided in disciplines, e.g. anatomy or physiology.

ADMISSIONS DATA

CHARACTERISTICS OF McMASTER MEDICAL STUDENTS AT ADMISSION

The Admissions policy of McMaster Medical School is broader than that of traditional medical schools. It places emphasis on the personal qualities of the students as well as their previous academic record and allows access to medical education by people from a wider range of academic backgrounds than is customary.

Some statistics on the students selected include:

(1) Twenty-four percent of the student body entering from 1969-1977 had an undergraduate grade point average (G.P.A.) below 3.00. Forty-eight percent had a G.P.A. between 3.00 and 3.49. The remaining 28 percent had G.P.A.'s of 3.5 or more on a four point scale.

(2) Twenty-eight percent entered medical school after completing a graduate degree.

(3) The student body has a diversity of undergraduate majors. Nine percent of the students had degrees in the arts or humanities. An additional 24 percent held degrees in one of the social sciences. Twenty-six percent held degrees in the biological sciences. Chemistry (8%); other natural sciences (23%) and other health related areas (10%) round out this picture.

(4) The proportion of women students admitted to the medical school has increased rapidly. Ten percent of the first class were women. In the recent past, nearly half of the entering class are women (1977: 42%; 1978: 44%; 1979: 55%).

(5) While the majority of students entering the program (1969-1979) are in the 21-25 age group (64%), 23 percent are 26-30 and 9 percent are 31-40. Four percent are in the 17-20 age group.

Part 1

Joseph Smith is a 67-year-old retired office worker. His wife died when he was 58 years old, and at age 60 he took early retirement. About a year and a half later he became depressed, lonely and discouraged and then improved with appropriate treatment.

For the last four years he has had pain in the calf of his legs on walking. Recently, he could walk only about 300 yards without being forced to stop. He lives alone and has increasing difficulty in getting to and from the supermarket where he shops.

Two weeks ago, he noticed that the tip of his right great toe was bluish in colour. This blueness has now extended until the whole terminal phalanx is involved. The tip of his toe has become black and a foul odour is present. Pulses cannot be detected at the ankle, but a pulse is detectable in the popliteal fossa.

Part 2

You refer him to a cardiovascular surgeon for further investigation and treatment. The decision is taken to amputate the leg above the knee and the situation is explained to Mr. Smith. The operation is performed without delay.

There is an initial good post-operative recovery, but two days after the operation he complains of pain and a tight feeling in the stump. His temperature is 38.8°C, pulse rate 120/min., respirations are 28/min., and he complains of thirst and nausea.

The surgeon removes the dressing to observe that the wound is reddened, swollen, and a sero-sanguinous fluid oozes from one end. There is a foul odour from the dressing. Palpation of the tissue surrounding the incision is painful and a crackling sensation is felt on firm pressure.

Part 3

A gram stain of the exudate shows a few white blood cells, large numbers of gram positive bacilli, and a few gram negative bacilli. Aerobically, the cultures grew Escherichia coli and anaerobically a heavy growth of Clostridium perfringens.

(continued)

He is treated with ampicillin (1 gram every 6 hours), penicillin (10,000,000 I.U. daily), polyvalent clostridial antitoxin (20 ml. b.i.d.) and debridement of all necrotic tissue. The infection is successfully controlled. After two further weeks, Mr. Smith is ready for discharge, but no discharge plans have been made.

You call the Amputee Program at the Chedoke-McMaster Centre and Mr. Smith is accepted for prosthesis fitting, training and rehabilitation.

You emphasize to the program staff the additional problems of hygiene and nutrition that you have noted previously and they agree to consider this.

The day before discharge, Mr. Smith is worried; he explains to you that his only living relative is a sister in England, that he has no friends, that he receives only the Old Age Pension plus $40 per month from his last job and that the lease expires on his apartment in 5 days.

ISSUES ACTUALLY EXPLORED BY A TUTORIAL GROUP

Discipline Areas		Issues
MORPHOLOGY	(M)*	Anatomy of lower limb (particularly arterial circulation)
PHYSIOLOGY	(M)	Mechanisms of calf pain
BEHAVIOUR	(M)	Coping with retirement
	(m)	Reactions to amputation
		o "grief" from missing limb o prospect of rehabilitation o economic implications
CLINICAL SKILLS	(m)	Examination of pulses
MICROBIOLOGY/INFECTIOUS DISEASE	(M)	Clostridium infections
		o pathogenesis o management

* (M) – MAJOR
  (m) – minor

(continued)

PLANNERS' ISSUES GUIDE
FOR HEALTH CARE PROBLEM: "JOSEPH SMITH"

(Phase I, 1979)

Note to students: The issues listed here are suggestions for potential
areas that might be explored. Use this list only as
a guide.

DISCIPLINE/AREA	
APPLIED HEALTH PROFESSIONS	Occupational therapy. Role of physiotherapists.
BEHAVIOURAL SCIENCES	Grief process, depression. Retirement as a life crisis. Psychological aspects of aging.
CELL BIOLOGY/ BIOCHEMISTRY	Glycolysis, TCA cycle, and oxidative phosphorylation related to energy production.
CLINICAL EPIDEMIOLOGY & BIOSTATISTICS	Role of self-care. Compliance. Incidence of peripheral vascular diseases. Incidence post-surgical infections. Correlations of peripheral vascular disease with lifestyle disorder.
COMMUNITY SERVICES, AGENCIES & INSTITUTIONS	The health care of the elderly.
GROWTH, AGING & DEVELOPMENT	Theories of aging. Tissue repair and recovery from surgery in aged. Goal identification in rehabilitation of aged people. Aging: physical, cognitive, and social aspects.

continued ...

DISCIPLINE/AREA	
HUMAN AND SOCIO-ECONOMIC VALUES	The care of the poor. Housing problems for the aged. Medical accountability regarding supportive therapy.
INFECTIOUS DISEASES/MICROBIOLOGY	Anaerobic bacteria: why foul odour in gangrene? Source of gas? Fever as a response to infection. Post-surgical infection. Toxins and antitoxins.
MORPHOLOGY	Anatomy of blood supply and lymph drainage of the lower limb. Peripheral circulation.
OCCUPATIONAL HEALTH	Why did the man retire? Was he given the right advice?
PATHOLOGY	The inflammatory reaction. Atheroma; gangrene.
PHARMACOLOGY	Drugs affecting the blood supply to tissues.
PHYSIOLOGY	Peripheral circulation. How is it normally regulated? Body temperature. What is the significance of the fever? Alternatively, how is it that body temperature is normally so constant?

Number of Irregular Events+

	'81	'80	'79	'78	'77	TOTAL
Remedial program due to "Unsatisfactory" evaluation	4	16 x	12 o	8	5 *	45
On Special Program "Flexibility"	0	1	2	5	0	8
Temporary Withdrawal						
(a) Leave of Absence	2	8	2	6	3	21
(b) Illness	1	2	2	–	–	5
Permanent Withdrawal						
(a) Dismissal from program for academic reasons	0	1	0	–	–	1
(b) Student initiated	0	1	0	1	3	5
TOTAL	7	29	18	20	11	85

+ There were 63 students who generated the 85 irregularities

x 10 students generated 16 "Unsatisfactory" evaluations

o 10 students generated 12 "Unsatisfactory" evaluations

*   3 students generated 5 "Unsatisfactory" evaluations

December 1979

CANADIAN INTERNSHIP MATCHING SERVICE RESULTS

1. 85% of McMaster students from 1972 to 1979 participated in the Match.

2. 77% of participating students received their first preference, compared to a national average of 65% receiving their first choice.

3. 97% of participating McMaster students were matched.

CIMS RESULTS: CLASS OF '80

PROGRAM	NUMBER OF STUDENTS		
	McMaster	Elsewhere	Total
MIXED INTERNSHIP	16	7	23
ROTATING INTERNSHIP	–	11	11
FAMILY MEDICINE	21	13	34
MEDICINE	5	10	15
SURGERY	4	1	5
PEDIATRICS	4	–	4
PSYCHIATRY	1	–	1
TOTAL	51	42	93
Not matched – 2			

LOCATION OF PROGRAM FOR 1980 GRADS

Hamilton	51
Toronto	18
Kingston	4
Montreal	4
Halifax	2
St. John's	1
Vancouver	4
Ottawa	1
London	5
Calgary	2
Victoria	1
TOTAL	93

145

1979 ANNUAL UPDATE OF McMASTER MEDICAL GRADUATES
SUMMARY & OBJECTIVES

This brief, yearly survey of all McMaster medical graduates is undertaken to establish their current location, function and specialty. This tracking study will allow ready identification of samples for future performance studies. It has also facilitated the development of an M.D. alumni chapter.

Summary of Results of Alumni Tracking Study for 1979

1. Overall direct response rate to this survey was 77%.
   Response rate increases as length of time from graduation increases.

2. Family Practice and General Practice are the career choices of 50% of McMaster M.D. graduates. Internal medicine attracts 18% of graduates.

3. The majority (62%) of McMaster medical alumni stay in Ontario. Of those that leave the province, 16% go to the United States, 13% choose western Canada, 6% locate in eastern Canada and the remaining 2% are scattered across the globe.

4. More than half of the graduates from 1976 to 1978 are still in training while 75% of 1972, 1973, and 1974 graduates are in practice.

5. Group practice is the most popular type of practice. (Forty percent of the graduates in practice chose group arrangements.)

6. Almost half of the first three classes of graduating students are now certified in family medicine or a specialty.

McMASTER MEDICAL SCHOOL PERFORMANCE
ON THE MEDICAL COUNCIL OF CANADA EXAMINATION

A Brief Overview

McMaster medical graduates' performance on the Medical Council of
Canada examination has varied from year to year. In 1979, McMaster
graduates performed above the national average in Part B of the Medical
Council of Canada examination. Only one student (1.1%) of 1979 graduates
failed both Part A and Part B. However, six students (6.6%) failed Part
A. Most of these failures were marginal (within a few points of the cut
off score).

One of the stable findings within Part A is that McMaster medical
graduates perform consistently well in the public health section relative
to their overall performance. Their peformance in the other clinical
disciplines tends to shift from year to year without a predictable
pattern emerging.

Part B of the Medical Council of Canada examination consists of
paper management problems, reviewing slides and x-rays, etc. It has a
problem-oriented focus. Part A of the examination consists entirely of
multiple choice questions. Some require problem-solving while others
emphasize factual recall. Except for one year, McMaster students have
performed relatively better on Part B than Part A.

Not all McMaster graduates chose to take the Medical Council of
Canada examination (2.1%) and/or take the examination at the time of
graduation (1.7%). Most of these students later successfully took the
examination. Some are studying in the United States and may have taken
FLEX or National Board examinations to obtain licensing. We are only
aware of licensing outside of Canada if the graduate chooses to reveal
this fact. Most of McMaster medical graduates who choose to become
licensed have. Only twelve graduates (2.6% of all graduates through
1978) who have taken the M.C.C. examination have not been licensed. More
than 97% of McMaster graduates (1972-1978) are licensed.

CANADIAN CERTIFICATION EXAMINATIONS PERFORMANCE

Summary of Objectives

This project monitors the performance of McMaster medical graduates who attempt one of the specialty certification examinations of the Royal College of Physicians and Surgeons or the certification examination in Family Medicine which is offered by the College of Family Physicians of Canada. The first time pass rate for both the written and oral examinations is documented as well as the number of graduates certified.

Summary of Results

Royal College of Physicians and Surgeons

1. Seventy-eight graduates have taken 90 written specialty certification examinations administered by the Royal College of Physicians and Surgeons. Their overall first time pass rate on the written portion is 85%.

2. The overall first time pass rate on the oral portion of a certification examination is 90%.

3. Four graduates are certified in two specialties. Eight additional graduates are working towards certification in two specialties.

4. Graduates are certified in sixteen different specialties recognized by the Royal College of Physicians and Surgeons. Internal Medicine (18 certified) and Pediatrics (10 certified) are the specialties with the largest number of certificands.

5. Forty-eight graduates have achieved specialty certification by the Royal College of Physicians and Surgeons. This is 17% of the first five graduating classes. (This figure under-represents the total number of graduates certified in a specialty. Some graduates have chosen to take only the U.S. specialty certification examinations.)

6. The total number of McMaster medical graduates certified by the RCPS has doubled in the past year. As of spring, 1979, 24 were certified; now 48 are certified. This reflects the growing number of graduates who are eligible for certification.

COLLEGE OF FAMILY PHYSICIANS OF CANADA (CFPC)

1. By 1979, 54 McMaster medical graduates were certified by the CFPC.

2. The overall first time pass rate on this examination is 95%.

A FOLLOW UP STUDY CURRENTLY UNDERWAY

CAREER CHOICES AND DEVELOPMENT OF McMASTER MEDICAL SCHOOL GRADUATES:
A SURVEY OF THE FIRST SIX GRADUATING CLASSES

Summary

As part of a longitudinal evaluation of the new medical school at
McMaster University, the first six graduating classes are surveyed using
mailed questionnaires to obtain information regarding their career
development, including postgraduate training experiences, career plans,
and location. An assessment of their undergraduate medical education by
the graduate physicians is included. The first three classes are
surveyed five years after graduation while the second three classes are
surveyed two years beyond graduation. This information will be useful to
both the medical school in monitoring the impact of its policies and to
the wider community concerned with the delivery of health care. The
impact of the new McMaster Medical School's graduates on the medical
manpower pool in Ontario and Canada will be ascertained.

Progress to Date

Data has been collected for the graduating classes of 1972 and 1973
five years after graduation and for the graduating classes of 1975 and
1976 two years after graduation. Ninety percent of the graduates
surveyed responded to the questionnaire.

Findings

Some preliminary findings include:

More than half of McMaster medical graduates (1972, 1973, 1975,
1976) chose straight internships. Fifty-eight percent (112) report
directly entering and completing residency training; twenty-eight (15%)
went directly into practice after their internship, while an additional
18 (9%) left a residency program to enter general practice. Seven (4%)
initially entered general practice and then returned for residency
training. Nearly one-quarter (23%) had decided on their medical field
before entering medical school; about one-third (34%) chose their
specialty while in medical school, while 29% did so as postgraduate
students. Ten percent indicate they are still undecided as to their
eventual field within medicine.

Although the proportion of men (43%) and women (45%) choosing
primary care is nearly equal, men are more likely to complete a family
medicine residency program (77%; 47 of 61; compared to 59%; 13 of 22)
than women while women are more likely than men to call themselves
general practitioners (41% to 23%, respectively). Men are also more
likely to enter subspecialty training in internal medicine (13%) than
women (6%).

Graduates in practice indicate they spend a median of 60 hours per week engaged in professional activities. Most frequently (45%) these graduates learned of the availability of their practice location while completing postgraduate training. The factors most often ranked among the three most important to the graduate in attracting them to their current practice locations included: (1) climate or geographic features of the area; (2) preference for urban or rural living; (3) influence of spouse; (4) opportunity to join a desirable partnership or group practice; (5) availability of clinical support facilities and personnel and (6) high medical need area. Factors (3) and (6) were ranked first most often. Thirty-four percent reported practicing in a small town or rural area.

McMaster medical graduates (1972, 1973, 1975 and 1976) also were asked about their undergraduate medical curriculum. One hundred fifty-four (81%) report that the three-year curriculum suited them. Overall 82% of these graduates felt the advantages of the three-year curriculum outweighed its disadvantages. The classes five years out (1972 = 100%; 1973 = 93%) are more likely to see the three-year curriculum as an advantage.

The class of 1975 reports the greatest number of disadvantages and only 73% feel the advantages of a three-year curriculum outweighed its disadvantages. This class is more negative in its program feedback than any other class (across items). The reasons for this are unclear. They were in medical school when student enrollment expanded rapidly. Only 31 (48%) said the McMaster medical program would appeal to them if they were beginning their medical school years again. Twenty percent of 1975 graduates felt less prepared for internship than other trainees they met. (Across the three other classes surveyed, only 9% felt less prepared for internship).

McMaster medical graduates felt as well or better prepared in most skill areas as compared with other students. The areas where at least 25% indicated they were less prepared are: therapeutic management; drug effects; basic science information and medical emergencies. Ninety-five percent (or more) of graduates indicated they felt well prepared in these areas: data gathering skills; problem-solving; social and emotional factors of illness; follow up medical care; self-evaluation techniques; behavioural science information and preparation for independent learning.

As mentioned earlier, the class of 1975 has a more negative program perception than other classes. This is also seen in the number of items they identify as program strengths and weaknesses. Two-thirds (or more) of the graduates surveyed identified the following features as program strengths: early patient contact; self-directed learning; small group tutorials; and independent study. Weaknesses identified by one-third or more of graduates are: anxiety level created and the evaluation system.

151

APPENDIX B

THE McMASTER M.D. PROGRAM:
TABLES

AGE AT ADMISSION TO McMASTER MEDICAL SCHOOL

(STUDENTS ENTERING BETWEEN 1969-1979)

Age Groups			
17-20	21-25	26-30	31-40
32 (4%)	553 (64%)	202 (23%)	78 (9%)

N = 865

Unknown 8

PREVIOUS ACADEMIC DEGREES OF McMASTER MEDICAL STUDENTS

(STUDENTS ENTERING 1969 - 1977)

Degrees Obtained	Number of Students	Percentage
Technical School Degree	10	1.5
Undergraduate Degree	656	98.4
Postgraduate Degree		
Masters	146)	27.8
Doctorate	39)) 185	

UNDERGRADUATE GRADE POINT AVERAGE OF

McMASTER MEDICAL STUDENTS

(STUDENTS ENTERING 1969-1977)

	Grade Point Average				
	<2.5	2.50-2.99	3.00-3.49	3.50-4.00	Total*
N	46	115	321	183	665
	7	17	48	28	100

* 7 missing values, G.P.A. could not be compared on 4 point scale.

UNDERGRADUATE ACADEMIC MAJOR OF McMASTER MEDICAL STUDENTS

(STUDENTS ENTERING 1969 - 1977)

Major	Year of Entry									Total	Percent
	69	70	71	72	73	74	75	76	77		
Chemistry	1	6	3	8	3	9	7	6	10	53	8
Biology	6	11	19	17	26	21	27	19	25	171	26
Other Natural Sciences	7	8	18	18	20	24	19	24	17	155	23
Psychology	2	6	9	13	13	11	17	21	14	106	16
Other Social Sciences	3	5	5	7	4	7	9	4	9	53	8
Arts and Humanities	1	3	5	11	12	5	8	12	6	63	9
Other Health Related	0	1	3	6	2	6	14	14	19	65	10
TOTAL	20	40	62	80	80	83	101	100	100	666	

Summary & Objectives

This brief, yearly survey of all McMaster medical graduates is undertaken to establish their current location, function and speciality. This tracking study will allow ready identification of samples for future performance studies. It has also facilitated the development of an M.D. alumni chapter.

Summary of Results of Alumni Tracking Study for 1979

(1) Overall direct response rate to this survey was 77%.
    Response rate increases as length of time from graduation increases.

(2) Family practice and general practice are the career choices of 50% of McMaster M.D. graduates. Internal medicine attracts 18% of graduates.

(3) The majority (62%) of McMaster medical alumni stay in Ontario. Of those that leave the province, 16% go to the United States, 13% choose western Canada, 6% locate in eastern Canada and the remaining 3% are scattered across the globe.

(4) More than half of the graduates from 1976 to 1978 are still in training while 75% of 1972, 1973, and 1974 graduates are in practice.

(5) Group practice is the most popular type of practice. (Forty percent of the graduates in practice chose group arrangements.)

(6) Almost half of the first three classes of graduating students are now certified in family medicine or a specialty.

PROPORTION OF MEN AND WOMEN BY GRADUATING YEAR

Graduating Year	Class Total	Men		Women	
		Number	%	Number	%
1972	19	17	89	2	10
1973	40	35	87	5	12
1974	68	53	78	15	22
1975	72	48	67	24	33
1976	82	56	68	26	32
1977	77	45	58	32	42
1978	102	51	50	51	50
1979	99	58	59	41	41
Total	559	363	65	196	35

1979 LOCATION OF ALL STUDENTS FROM THE M.D. GRADUATING CLASSES OF 1972 THROUGH 1978

CLASS	ONTARIO		EASTERN CANADA		WESTERN CANADA		U.S.A.		ELSEWHERE		TOTAL		BOTH MALE & FEMALE
	MALE	FEMALE	MALE	FEMALE	MALE	FEMALE	MALE	FEMALE	MALE	FEMALE	MALE	FEMALE	
1972	7	2	1	-	1	-	6	-	2	-	17	2	19
1973	20	2	1	2	3	1	9	-	2	-	35	5	40
1974	28	7	1	2	8	2	12	3	4	1	53	15	68
1975	25	14	3	1	9	4	11	4	1	-	49	23	72
1976	36	11	-	5	9	7	8	4	2	-	55	27	82
1977	31	25	1	1	4	1	8	6	-	-	44	33	77
1978	41	36	3	7	5	5	3	1	-	-	52	49	101
TOTAL	188 (62)	97 (63)	10 (3)	18 (12)	39 (13)	20 (13)	57 (19)	18 (12)	11 (4)	12 (3)	305 (66)	154 (34)	459
# AND % OF GRADUATED STUDENTS IN VARIOUS LOCATIONS	285 (62)		28 (6)		59 (13)		75 (16)		12 (3)		459		TOTAL n FROM CLASSES '72 THROUGH '78

TOTAL # OF GRADUATES

- IN CANADA = 372
- IN U.S.A. = 75
- ELSEWHERE = 12

PERCENTAGES (in brackets) represent the percentage of each sex in each location.
WESTERN CANADA includes Manitoba, Saskatchewan, Alberta, B.C., Yukon and N.W.T.
EASTERN CANADA includes Quebec, Maritimes and Newfoundland.
ELSEWHERE includes Angola, Australia, Zambia, New Zealand, Saudi Arabia, Scotland, Sierra Leone, Tanzania, Western Samoa, and Papua New Guinea.

LOCATION OF McMASTER M.D. GRADUATES CURRENTLY "IN TRAINING"

Alberta	6
British Columbia	13
Manitoba	5
Nova Scotia	2
Newfoundland	2
Ontario	221
Quebec	22
Saskatchewan	1
TOTAL IN CANADA	272
United States of America	41
Other*	5
TOTAL IN TRAINING	318

*   Includes graduates located in Australia (2), New Zealand, Scotland and Tanzania.

LOCATION OF McMASTER M.D. GRADUATES CURRENTLY "IN PRACTICE"

Alberta	3
British Columbia	28
Newfoundland/Labrador	2
Manitoba	4
Ontario	136
Prince Edward Island	2
Quebec	5
Saskatchewan	1
Nova Scotia	2
Yukon Territory	3
TOTAL IN CANADA	185
United States of America	41
Other*	8
TOTAL IN PRACTICE	235**

*   Includes graduates located in Angola, Australia,
New Guinea, Saudi Arabia, Sierra Leone,
West Germany, Western Samoa and Xambia.

**   Unable to certify current status on five graduates.

CURRENT LEVEL OF THOSE GRADUATES IN TRAINING (AUGUST 1979)

LEVEL OF TRAINING	1972	1973	1974	1975	1976	1977	1978	TOTAL MALES	TOTAL FEMALES	GRAND TOTAL
INTERN	-	-	-	-	-	1 (2)	8 (9)	5 (4)	4 (5)	9 (4)
RESIDENT 1	-	-	1 (6)	-	1 (3)	4 (10)	26 (30)	18 (13)	14 (17)	32 (15)
RESIDENT 2	-	-	-	3 (10)	4 (10)	19 (46)	50 (58)	39 (29)	37 (45)	76 (34)
RESIDENT 3	-	-	1 (6)	3 (10)	11 (28)	14 (34)	1 (1)	19 (14)	11 (13)	30 (14)
RESIDENT 4	-	1 (17)	1 (6)	5 (16)	15 (38)	1 (2)	-	17 (13)	6 (7)	23 (10)
RESIDENT 5	1 (100)	1 (17)	2 (13)	5 (16)	-	-	-	9 (7)		9 (4)
RESIDENT 6	-	1 (17)	1 (6)	-	-	-	-	1		2 (1)
CHIEF RESIDENT	-	1 (17)	1 (6)	5 (16)	3 (8)	-	-	7 (5)	3 (4)	10 (5)
TEACHING FELLOW	-	-	1 (6)	2 (7)	-	1 (2)	-	1 (1)	3 (4)	4 (2)
RESEARCH FELLOW	-	1 (17)	4 (25)	5 (16)	5 (13)	-	1 (1)	14 (10)	2 (2)	16 (7)
GRADUATE STUDENT	-	1 (17)	2 (13)	1 (3)	1 (3)	-	-	5 (2)	2 (2)	7 (2)
OTHER	-	-	2 (13)	1 (3)	-	-	-	3 (2)	-	3 (1)
UNKNOWN	-	-	-	1 (3)	-	-	-	-	1 (1)	1 (.5)
TOTAL IN TRAINING	1	6	16	31	40	40	86	138	85	223

THERE ARE 2 M.D. GRADUATES THAT ARE NOT INDICATED ON THIS TABLE. ONE '76 GRADUATE IS CURRENTLY DOING A PH.D. IN BIOPHYSICS. ONE '77 GRADUATE IS IN DENTAL SCHOOL FULL TIME. BOTH ARE PHYSICIANS PART TIME.

164

PROPORTION OF McMASTER GRADUATES IN PRACTICE AND IN TRAINING (AS OF AUGUST 1979)
(1972-1978 GRADUATES)

	1972	1973	1974	1975	1976	1977	1978	TOTAL MALE	TOTAL FEMALE	GRAND TOTAL
IN PRACTICE	18 (95)	34 (85)	50 (74)	41 (57)	39 (48)	36 (47)	14 (14)	166 (54)	66 (43)	232 (50)
IN TRAINING	1 (5)	6 (15)	16 (24)	31 (43)	40 (49)	40 (52)	86 (84)	136 (44)	84 (55)	220 (48)
TRAVELLING & TIME OFF			1 (1)		1 (1)		1 (1)	1 (.3)	2 (1)	3 (1)
UNLOCATABLE			1 (1)		2 (2)	1 (1)	1 (1)	3 (1)	2 (1)	5 (1)
TOTAL	19	40	68	72	82	77	102	306	154	460

Numbers shown in (brackets) are percentages of column totals.

165

SPECIALTY CHOICE OF McMASTER M.D. GRADUATES

SPECIALTY CHOICE	AS REPORTED IN 1977	AS REPORTED IN 1978	AS REPORTED IN 1979
+ FAMILY MEDICINE	76 (27%)	91 (31%)	135 (29%)
+ GENERAL PRACTICE	56 (20%)	44 (15%)	97 (21%)
* INTERNAL MEDICINE	59 (21%)	60 (20%)	83 (18%)
** SURGERY	24 (9%)	22 (8%)	39 (9%)
PSYCHIATRY	15 (5%)	15 (5%)	33 (7%)
*** PEDIATRICS	18 (6%)	14 (4%)	21 (5%)
OBSTETRICS/GYNECOLOGY	10 (4%)	7 (2%)	12 (3%)
****OTHER	20 (7%)	40 (14%)	35 (8%)
UNKNOWN	3 (1%)	3 (1%)	5 (1%)
TOTAL	281	296	460

* MEDICINE INCLUDES – CARDIOLOGY, CLINICAL IMMUNOLOGY, DERMATOLOGY, GASTROENTEROLOGY, HEMATOLOGY, INTERNAL MEDICINE, NEUROLOGY, PHYSICAL MEDICINE AND REHABILITATION, RESPIRATORY MEDICINE, RHEUMATOLOGY.

** SURGERY INCLUDES – CARDIOVASCULAR AND THORACIC SURGERY, GENERAL SURGERY, NEUROSURGERY, OPHTHALMOLOGY, ORTHOPEDIC SURGERY, OTOLARYNGOLOGY, PLASTIC SURGERY, UROLOGY.

*** PEDIATRICS INCLUDES – PEDIATRIC CARDIOLOGY, PEDIATRIC GENERAL SURGERY, PEDIATRICS.

****OTHER INCLUDES – ANAESTHESIA, ANATOMICAL PATHOLOGY, COMMUNITY MEDICINE, DIAGNOSTIC RADIOLOGY, GENERAL PATHOLOGY, HEMATOLOGICAL PATHOLOGY, MEDICAL BIOCHEMISTRY, MEDICAL MICROBIOLOGY, NEUROPATHOLOGY, NUCLEAR MEDICINE, RADIATION ONCOLOGY, EMERGENCY MEDICINE, EPIDEMIOLOGY AND OTHERS.

+ SELF REPORT IS USED FOR THIS CATEGORIZATION.

SPECIALTY CHOICE OF McMASTER M.D. GRADUATES – CLASSES OF 1972 THROUGH 1978

	1972	1973	1974	1975	1976	1977	1978	TOTAL
PRIMARY CARE*	9/19 (47%)	23/40 (58%)	36/68 (53%)	39/72 (54%)	40/82 (49%)	42/77 (55%)	55/102 (54%)	244/460 (53%)
OTHER SPECIALTIES	10/19 (53%)	17/40 (42%)	31/68 (46%)	33/72 (46%)	41/82 (50%)	33/77 (43%)	46/102 (45%)	211/460 (46%)
UNKNOWN			1/68 (1%)		1/82 (1%)	2/77 (2%)	1/102 (1%)	5/460 (1%)

*Includes graduates indicating specialty choice of Family Medicine, General Practice and Emergency Medicine.

167

PERCENTAGE OF McMASTER M.D. GRADUATES IN "PRIMARY CARE"
AS REPORTED IN THE 1979 ANNUAL UPDATE, BY YEAR OF GRADUATION

Year	Number	Percent
1972	9	47
1973	23	58
1974	36	53
1975	39	54
1976	40	49
1977	41	53
1978	55	54
TOTAL	243	53

SPECIALTY CHOICE BY GRADUATING YEAR (1972 - 1978 GRADUATES)

SPECIALTY	1972	1973	1974	1975	1976	1977	1978	TOTAL MALES	TOTAL FEMALES	GRAND TOTAL
ANAESTHESIA	1 (5)	-	1 (2)	-	1 (1)	3 (4)	-	5 (2)	1 (.6)	6 (1)
ANATOMIC PATHOLOGY	-	-	-	1 (1)	-	-	-	1 (.3)		1 (.2)
CARDIOLOGY	-	-	2 (3)	2 (3)	4 (5)	-	-	8 (3)		8 (2)
CARDIOVASCULAR THORACIC SURGERY	-	2 (5)	-	-	-	-	-	2 (1)		2 (.4)
CLINICAL IMMUNOLOGY						1 (1)	-		1 (.6)	1 (.2)
COMMUNITY MEDICINE						1 (1)	-		1 (.6)	1 (.2)
DERMATOLOGY	1 (5)	-	-	4 (6)	-	1 (1)	-	5 (2)	1 (.6)	6 (1)
DIAGNOSTIC RADIOLOGY	-	-	-	1 (1)	1 (1)	-	-	2 (1)		2 (.4)
GASTROENTEROLOGY	-	-	-	1 (1)	-	-	-	1 (.3)		1 (.2)
GENERAL PATHOLOGY	-	-	-	1 (1)	-	-	-	1 (.3)		1 (.2)
GENERAL SURGERY	1 (5)	-	1 (2)	1 (1)	2 (2)	2 (3)	3 (3)	9 (3)	1 (.6)	10 (2)
HEMATOLOGY	1 (5)	-	1 (2)	-	-	-	-	2 (1)		2 (.4)
INTERNAL MEDICINE	1 (5)	2 (5)	6 (9)	5 (7)	8 (10)	8 (10)	14 (14)	31 (10)	13 (8)	44 (10)
MEDICAL BIOCHEMISTRY	-	-	-	-	-	-	1 (1)	-	1 (.6)	1 (.2)
NEUROLOGY	1 (5)	-	3 (4)	2 (3)	-	1 (1)	-	4 (1)	3 (2)	7 (2)
NEUROSURGERY	-	-	-	-	-	1 (1)	1 (1)	2 (1)		2 (.4)
NUCLEAR MEDICINE	-	-	-	1 (1)	-	-	-	1 (.3)		1 (.2)
OBSTETRICS & GYNECOLOGY	1 (5)	1 (3)	4 (6)	-	3 (4)	1 (1)	2 (2)	8 (3)	4 (3)	12 (3)
OPHTHALMOLOGY	-	2 (5)	-	1 (1)	3 (4)	1 (1)	4 (4)	7 (2)	4 (3)	11 (2)

SPECIALITY CHOICE BY GRADUATING YEAR (continued)

ORTHOPEDIC SURGERY	-	-	1 (2)	1 (1)	3 (4)	1 (1)	2 (2)	7 (2)	1 (.6)	8 (2)
OTOLARYNGOLOGY	-	-	1 (2)	-	-	-	1 (1)	2 (1)		2 (.4)
PEDIATRICS	1 (5)	4 (10)	2 (3)	3 (4)	2 (2)	4 (5)	5 (5)	12 (4)	9 (6)	21 (5)
PHYSICAL MEDICINE & REHABILITATION	1 (5)	-	1 (2)	-	-	1 (1)	2 (2)	4 (1)	1 (.6)	5 (1)
PLASTIC SURGERY	-	-	1 (2)	-	2 (2)	-	-	2 (1)	1 (.6)	3 (1)
PSYCHIATRY	-	3 (8)	2 (3)	5 (7)	8 (10)	5 (7)	10 (10)	19 (6)	14 (9)	33 (7)
RADIATION ONCOLOGY	-	1 (3)	-	-	-	-	-	1 (.3)		1 (.2)
RESPIRATORY MEDICINE	1 (5)	-	-	2 (3)	1 (1)	1 (1)	-	5 (2)		5 (1)
RHEUMATOLOGY	-	1 (3)	2 (3)	-	1 (1)	-	-	3 (1)	1 (.6)	4 (1)
UROLOGY	-	-	-	1 (1)	-	-	-	1 (.3)		1 (.2)
EMERGENCY MEDICINE	1 (5)	1 (3)	1 (2)	2 (3)	4 (5)	3 (4)	-	10 (3)	2 (1)	12 (3)
FAMILY MEDICINE	4 (21)	16 (40)	19 (28)	16 (22)	20 (24)	24 (31)	36 (35)	85 (28)	50 (33)	135 (29)
GENERAL PRACTICE	4 (21)	.6 (15)	16 (24)	21 (29)	16 (20)	15 (19)	19 (19)	60 (20)	37 (24)	97 (21)
OTHER	-	-	1 (2)	1 (1)	1 (1)	-	1 (1)	2 (.7)	2 (1)	4 (1)
EPIDEMIOLOGY	-	1 (3)	2 (3)	-	1 (1)	1 (1)	-	2 (.7)	3 (2)	5 (1)
UNKNOWN	-	-	1 (2)	-	1 (1)	2 (3)	1 (1)	2 (.7)	3 (2)	5 (1)
TOTAL	19 (4)	40 (9)	68 (15)	72 (16)	82 (18)	77 (17)	102(22)	306	154	460

Numbers in (brackets) are percentages.

TOTAL percentages are row percentages and all others are column percentages.

TYPE OF PRACTICE	1972	1973	1974	1975	1976	1977	1978	TOTAL MALE	TOTAL FEMALE	GRAND TOTAL
SOLO	5 (28)	13 (38)	14 (28)	13 (32)	12 (31)	13 (36)	1 (7)	52 (31)	19 (29)	71 (31)
GROUP	9 (50)	15 (44)	22 (44)	19 (46)	14 (36)	10 (28)	4 (29)	70 (42)	22 (33)	92 (40)
INSTITUTION – GOVERNMENT, UNIVERSITY, ETC.	3 (17)	4 (12)	8 (16)	8 (20)	11 (28)	7 (19)	3 (21)	28 (17)	16 (24)	44 (19)
OTHER	1 (6)	2 (6)	6 (12)	1 (2)	2 (5)	6 (17)	6 (43)	16 (10)	9 (14)	25 (11)
TOTAL IN PRACTICE	18	34	50	41	39	36	14	166	66	232

Numbers shown in (brackets) are percentages of column totals.

171

McMASTER MEDICAL SCHOOL PERFORMANCE
ON THE MEDICAL COUNCIL OF CANADA EXAMINATION

A Brief Overview

McMaster medical graduates' performance on the Medical Council of Canada examination has varied from year to year. Table 1 presents the scaled (adjusted) score for Part A and Part B of the examination by year. As you will note, the national rank varies from 3 to 15 in Part A and 1 to 11 in Part B. However, minor differences in score can cause significant shifts in rank as most schools' scores are within two or three points of each other. Thus, in 1979, the Medical Council discontinued the use of ranks.

In 1979, McMaster graduates performed above the national average in Part B of the Medical Council of Canada examination (see Table 1). Only one student (1.1% of 1979 McMaster graduates sitting the examination) failed Part B. None of the 1979 graduates failed both Part A and Part B (see Table 2). However, six students (6.6%) failed Part A. Most of these failures were marginal (within a few points of the cut-off score).

One of the stable findings within Part A is that McMaster medical graduates perform consistently well in the public health section relative to their overall performance. Their performance in the other clinical disciplines tends to shift from year to year without a predictable pattern emerging.

Part B of the Medical Council of Canada examination consists of paper management problems, reviewing slides and x-rays, etc. It has a problem-oriented focus. Part A of the examination consists entirely of multiple choice questions. Some require problem-solving while other emphasize factual recall. Except for one year, McMaster students have performed relatively better on Part B than Part A (see Table 1).

Not all McMaster graduates chose to take the Medical Council of Canada examination and/or take the examination at the time of graduation (See Table 3). Most of these students later successfully take the examination. Some are studying in the United States and may have taken FLEX or National Board examinations to obtain licensing. We are only aware of licensing outside of Canada if the graduate chooses to reveal this fact. Most of McMaster medical graduates who choose to become licensed have. Only twelve graduates (2.6% of graduates through 1978) who have taken the M.C.C. examination have not been licensed. More than 97% of McMaster graduates (1972-1978) are licensed.

McMASTER MEDICAL SCHOOL
MCC PERFORMANCE 1972-1979

	Part A	Part B	National Rank A	B
1972	74 (71)*	75 (71)	3	1
1973	68 (68)	69 (69)	11	10
1974	70 (69)	70 (69)	7	7
1975	69 (69)	70 (69)	11	6
1976	69 (69)	72 (69)	12	2
1977	69 (69)	69 (69)	7	10
1978	67 (69)	68 (69)	15	11
1979	67 (69)	69 (68)	--	--

* Figures in brackets are the
  national average that year.

McMASTER MEDICAL SCHOOL
MEDICAL COUNCIL OF CANADA EXAMINATION PERFORMANCE*

Grad. Yr.	PART A Pass	Fail	PART B Pass	Fail	OVERALL Pass	Fail	N
1972	19 (100)	0	19 (100)	0	19 (100)	0	19
1973+	39 (97.5)	1 (2)	35 (87.5)	5 (12)	35 (87.5)	5 (12)	40
1974+	67 (98.5)	1 (2)	63 (92.6)	5 (7)	63 (92.6)	5 (7)	68
1975v	66 (93.0)	5 (7)	67 (94.4)	4 (6)	65 (91.6)	6 (8)	71
1976o	66 (91.7)	6 (8)	68 (94.5)	4 (5)	64 (88.9)	8 (11)	72
1977o	73 (87.3)	2 (3)	70 (93.3)	5 (7)	70 (93.3)	5 (7)	75
1978-	93 (94.9)	5 (5)	90 (91.8)	8 (8)	89 (91.8)	9 (9)	98
1979	85 (93.3)	6 (7)	90 (98.9)	1 (1)	84 (92.3)	7 (8)	91
Over-all Total	508 (95)	26 (5)	502 (94)	32 (6)	489 (92)	45 (8)	534

( ) Percentage

+   1 student failed Part A & B

o   2 students failed Part A & B

v   3 students failed Part A & B

−   4 students failed Part A & B

*   For students who took the examination in their graduation year, first attempt only. McMaster Medical School has graduated 556 students. Ninety-six graduated in 1979.

OVERALL PERFORMANCE OF McMASTER MEDICAL GRADUATES
ON THE CANADIAN LICENSING EXAMINATION

Grad Year	Percentage of Graduated Class Known to Pass Licensing Examination	Class Size	Took MCC In Graduating Year	Pass 1st Attempt	Eventual Pass	No Pass+	No Attempts
1972	100%	19	19	19	0	0	0
1973	100%	40	40	35	4	1*	0
1974	98.6%	69	68	63	5	0	1
1975	94.4%	72	71	65	3	3	1
1976	92%	82	72	64 (3)	5 (3)	3 (1)	3
1977	97.4%	77	75	70 (1)	4	1	1
1978	95%	101	98	89 (2)	5	4	1
1979o	88%	96	91	84	NA	7	5

( ) First attempt not in grad year

* Pass U.S. Licensing examination

+ May have attempted and/or passed U.S. examination

o Have had only one opportunity to sit the examination

175

CANADIAN CERTIFICATION EXAMINATIONS PERFORMANCE

Summary of Objectives

This project monitors the performance of McMaster medical graduates who attempt one of the specialty certification examinations of the Royal College of Physicians and Surgeons or the certification examination in Family Medicine which is offered by the College of Family Physicians of Canada. The first time pass rate for both the written and oral examinations is documented as well as the number of graduates certified.

The performance of graduates on particular specialty examinations will be assessed as data accumulates.

McMASTER MEDICAL GRADUATES
CERTIFIED IN A SPECIALTY BY THE
ROYAL COLLEGE OF PHYSICIANS AND SURGEONS

Year of Graduation	Certified as of Feb. 1979		Certified as of Feb. 1980		Total Class Size
	N	%	N	%	
1972	7	37	7	37	19
1973	6	15	7	18	40
1974	11	16	19	28	68+
1975	--	--	13	18	72
1976	--	--	2	2	82
TOTAL	24	8	48	17	281

+ One graduate has died and is not included in the totals.

McMASTER MEDICAL GRADUATES CERTIFIED BY THE
COLLEGE OF FAMILY PHYSICIANS OF CANADA (CFPC)
OR THE ROYAL COLLEGE OF PHYSICIANS AND SURGEONS (RCPS)

Year of Graduation	CFPC+	RCPS[0]	Total Holding Canadian Certification	% of Class
1972	2	7	9	(47)
1973	9	7	16	(40)
1974	14	19	33	(48)
1975	5	13	18	(25)
1976	10	2	12	(15)
1977	14	--	14	
	54	48	102	

+   Updated summer 1979

0   Updated winter 1980

COMPARISON OF McMASTER MEDICAL STUDENTS AND OTHER CANADIAN MEDICAL SCHOOLS
CANADIAN INTERN MATCHING SERVICE RESULTS

	Total Graduates	Net # of Students Participating		Participating Students Receiving First Preference		# of Students Matched	
		N	% of total	N	% of participants	N	% of students participating
1972 – McMaster	19	16	84.2	15	93.8	16	100.00
– Other Canadian	803	585	72.8	446	55.5	567	96.9
1973 – McMaster	40	34	85.0	28	82.3	34	100.00
– Other Canadian	978	636	65.0	488	76.7	613	96.4
1974 – McMaster	69	66	95.6	49	74.2	62	93.9
– Other Canadian	1060	811	76.5	609	75.1	787	97.0
1975 – McMaster	77	63	81.8	50	79.4	59	93.7
– Other Canadian	1165	918	78.8	585	63.7	848	92.4
*1976 – McMaster	93	75	80.6	50	66.7	70	93.3
– Other Canadian	1315	1042	79.2	662	63.5	965	92.6
1977 – McMaster	85	67	78.8	47	70.2	66	98.5
– Other Canadian	1276	990	77.6	622	62.8	960	97.0
*1978 – McMaster	111	95	85.6	69	72.6	92	96.8
– Other Canadian	1292	1032	79.9	616	59.7	997	96.6
*1979 – McMaster	102	88	86.3	68	77.2	87	98.9
– Other Canadian	1305	1032	79.1	622	60.3	1007	97.6

* Total graduates includes graduates and graduating students.

CAREER CHOICES AND DEVELOPMENT OF McMASTER MEDICAL SCHOOL GRADUATES: A SURVEY OF THE FIRST SIX GRADUATING CLASSES

Summary

As part of the longitudinal evaluation of the new medical school at McMaster University, the first six graduating classes are surveyed using mailed questionnaires to obtain information regarding their career development, including postgraduate training experiences, career plans, and location. An assessment of their undergraduate medical education by the graduate physicians is included. The first three classes are surveyed five years after graduation while the second three classes are surveyed two years beyond graduation. This information will be useful to both the medical school in monitoring the impact of its policies and to the wider community concerned with the delivery of health care. The impact of the new McMaster Medical School's graduates on the medical manpower pool in Ontario and Canada will be ascertained.

Objectives

1)   To characterize the postgraduate training, career choices and practice preferences of McMaster Medical School graduates.

2)   To examine developmental trends in career choice and preference from medical school entry through entering practice and to isolate factors related to stability and shifts in career choice and practice preference.

3)   To examine the relationships among career path chosen, data obtained on admission (GPA; type of academic background, etc.) and performance during the medical program.

4)   To assess the extent to which career choice and practice location is related to stable socio-demographic information known at admission (e.g. age, sex, size of home town, etc.).

5)   To obtain an evaluation of the undergraduate medical training at McMaster University, in terms of its perceived relevance for the present activities of the first six graduating classes, and the extent to which it influenced decisions about career.

Major Questions

(a) Questions related to the admissions policies of the McMaster Medical School

   1. Do graduates who lacked the normal prerequisites to enter medical training differ from their classmates in career development subsequent to medical school on the following:

      a. Proportion changing career choice from program entry to two or five years after graduation
      b. Percentage choosing mixed, straight and rotating internships
      c. Percentage distribution among the various specialties
      d. Percentage distribution among practice setting (location and organization of practice)
      e. Intention to seek certification (2 years out) or proportion certified (5 years out)
      f. Significant factors in career choice, location (or intended location) of practice, and/or type of practice organization
      g. Their perceptions of the undergraduate medical program

   2. Do women graduates differ from their male classmates on these parameters? (Given in 1.a − 1.g)

   3. Do graduates over age 30 at time of entry differ from their classmates on these parameters?

   4. Are graduates with academic preparation (beyond bachelor's degree) and work experience in another field likely to combine these interests with their medical career?

(b) Questions related to the innovative medical curriculum

   1. Is there consistency across classes in the major strengths and weaknesses of the program as perceived by the graduates?

   2. What proportion of graduates felt well prepared for internship training?

   3. What educational skills and experiences acquired in the program have been useful in postgraduate experience?

(c) Questions related to broader issues in medical education

   1. Are women medical graduates today more likely than men to choose work situations with regular hours or flexible hours?

180

2. Are women medical graduates more likely than men to be over-represented in specialties which have attracted women in medicine in the past?

3. Is the size of home town of graduate related to practice location?

4. Does the size of home town of the spouse exert an influence on the size of community chosen for practice? Are men and women graduates different in this respect?

5. What are the preceived advantages of receiving an M.D. after three years of training rather than four years? What are the preceived disadvantages? Does prior academic background (G.P.A., courses chosen) influence these perceptions?

6. Are the benefits of a three-year medical curriculum seen as greater than its disadvantages by its graduates?

Current Status

The final year of data collection is now in progress. Overall response rate for the Classes of 1972, 1973, 1975 and 1976 was 90 percent. Response rate from the Classes of 1974 and 1977 currently stands at 76 percent. Two progress reports have been submitted to the granting agency (November 1, 1978 and November 1, 1979).

Funded by: The Ontario Ministry of Health

TIMETABLE

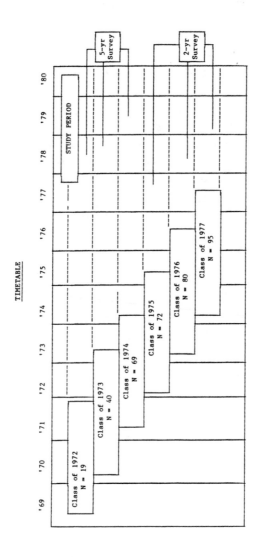

RESPONSE RATE TO SURVEY BY SEX AND YEAR OF GRADUATION

Sex \ Grad Year	1972		1973		1975		1976		TOTAL	
	N	%	N	%	N	%	N	%	N	%
MALE	17	(100)	30	(86)	46	(96)	50	(89)	143	(92)
FEMALE	2	(100)	5	(100)	19	(79)	23	(88)	49	(86)
TOTAL	19	(100)	35	(88)	65	(90)	73	(89)	192	(90)
CLASS SIZE	19		40		72		82		213	

% reflects percentage of entire graduated class

183

TABLES ILLUSTRATING CAREER PATHS AND DECISIONS

(1972, 1973, 1975, 1976)

WHAT TYPE OF INTERNSHIP OR FIRST YEAR RESIDENCY DID YOU TAKE?

Type of Internship \ Grad Yr	1972	1973	1975	1976	Total
Rotating	3 (16)*	14 (40)	7 (11)	22 (30)	46 (24)
Straight	14 (74)	15 (43)	39 (60)	37 (50)	104 (55)
Mixed	2 (10)	2 (6)	13 (20)	7 (10)	24 (12)
Other	0	4 (11)	6 (9)	7 (10)	17 (9)
TOTAL	19	35	65	73	192 (100)

* Percentages are given in brackets.

WHICH OF THE FOLLOWING STATEMENTS BEST DESCRIBES YOUR CAREER SINCE GRADUATION OR COMPLETING YOUR INTERNSHIP?

Career Since Graduation \ Grad Yr	1972	1973	1975	1976	Total
Entered and Remained in General Practice	4	5	11	8	28 (15%)
Entered General Practice and Left for a Residency Program	1	1	2	3	7 (4%)
Entered Residency and Left to Become a General Practitioner	1	4	8	5	18 (9%)
Entered and Completed or Completing Residency	6	23	36	47	112 (58%)
Other	7	2	8	10	27 (14%)
Total	19	35	65	73	192 (100%

RANK FACTORS IMPORTANT IN ATTRACTING YOU TO PRESENT LOCATION.

	First		Second		Third		N	Overall Rank
	N	%	N	%	N	%		
Climate or geographic features of area	10	9.3	19	18.3	10	10.6	39	1
Preference for urban or rural living	12	11	14	13.5	9	9.6	35	2
Influence of wife or husband (her/his desires, career, etc.)	15	14	7	6.7	1	1.1	23	3.5
Opportunity to join desirable partnership or group practice	9	8.4	7	6.7	7	7.4	23	3.5
Availability of clinical support facilities and personnel	4	3.7	9	8.7	8	8.5	21	5
High medical need in area	14	13	1	1.0	5	5.3	20	6
Income potential	4	3.7	11	5.7	4	4.3	19	7
Recreational and sports facilities	7	6.5	3	2.9	8	8.5	18	8
Opportunity for regular contact with a medical school or medical centre	6	5.6	4	3.8	6	6.4	16	9
Proximity to family of orgin	4	3.7	7	6.7	3	3.2	14	10
Opportunity for regular contact with other physicians	1	.9	3	2.9	9	9.6	13	11
Cultural advantages	1	.9	2	1.9	8	8.5	11	12.5
Recruited by colleagues	4	37	5	4.8	2	2.1	11	12.5
Having gone through medical school, internship and/or residency near here (circle all that apply)	3	3	2	1.9	3	3.2	8	14
Having been brought up in such a community	1	.9	4	3.8	2	2.1	7	15
Opportunities for social life	3	2.8	1	1.0	1	1.1	5	16.5
Prospect for being more influential in community affairs	1	.9	1	1.0	3	3.2	5	16.5
Loan payment	2	2	2	2.19			4	17
Availability of good social service, welfare or home care services	1	.9			1	1.1	2	19
Quality of educational system for children					2	2.1	2	19
Other			2	1.9	2	2.1	2	19
Organized efforts of community to recruit physicians	1	1					1	21
	(N = 107)		(N = 104)		(N = 94)			

107 are in practice and completed this item

PLEASE INDICATE THE SIZE OF MUNICIPALITY IN WHICH YOUR PRACTICE IS LOCATED

Community Size \ Grad Yr	1972	1973	1975	1976	TOTAL
Metropolitan Area 100,000	9 (56)*	20 (84)	18 (58)	8 (27)	55 (51)
Suburb of Metropolitan Area	0	0	1 (3)	1 (3)	2 (2)
Medium Sized City	1 (6)	2 (7)	5 (16)	5 (17)	13 (12)
Medium Sized Suburb	0	0	1 (3)	0	1 (1)
Town	5 (32)	5 (16)	1 (3)	9 (30)	20 (18)
Rural Area	1 (6)	4 (13)	5 (16)	7 (23)	17 (16)
Total	16 (100)	31 (100)	31 (100)	30 (100)	108

Missing Observations = 2 (73 + 76)

* Percentages are given in brackets

WHICH OF THE FOLLOWING STATEMENTS BEST DESCRIBES YOUR REACTION TO THE
COMPLETION OF YOUR UNDERGRADUATE MEDICAL EDUCATION IN THREE YEARS RATHER THAN
FOUR YEARS?

Reaction to 3 Year Program / Grad Yr	1972	1973	1975	1976	TOTAL
Suited	18 (95)*	29 (83)	49 (77)	58 (81)	154 (81)
Prefer 4 Years	0	2 (6)	1 (2)	3 (4)	6 (3)
4 Years with Added Experience	0	2 (6)	14 (22)	9 (12)	25 (13)
3 Years with Vacation	1 (5)	0	0	0	1 (.5)
Other	0	1 (3)	0	0	1 (.5)
Not Complete in 3 Years		1 (3)		2 (3)	3 (1)
Total	19 (10)	35 (18)	64 (34)	73 (38)	190

Missing Observations = 2

* Percentages are given in brackets

TABLES ILLUSTRATING PROGRAM FEEDBACK

NUMBER OF ADVANTAGES IN COMPLETING THE M.D. PROGRAM IN THREE YEARS

Number of Advantages \ Grad Yr	1972	1973	1975	1976	Total
None	1 (5)*	4 (12)	6 (9)	9 (13)	30 (11)
One	13 (69)	22 (67)	37 (57)	35 (51)	107 (57)
Two	5 (26)	6 (18)	20 (31)	21 (30)	52 (28)
Three	0	1 (3)	3 (3)	5 (6)	7 (4)
Total	19	33	65	69	186 (100)

Missing Observations = 6

NUMBER OF DISADVANTAGES OF COMPLETING THE M.D. PROGRAM IN THREE YEARS

Number of Disadvantages \ Grad Yr	1972	1973	1975	1976	Total
None	9 (47)	16 (50)	29 (44)	19 (28)	73 (40)
One	10 (53)	13 (41)	29 (44)	32 (46)	84 (45)
Two	0	2 (6)	5 (8)	15 (22)	22 (12)
Three	0		2 (3)	3 (4)	5 (3)
Five	0	1 (3)		0	1 (.5)
Total	19	32	65	69	185 (100)

Missing Observations = 7

OVERALL, DO THE ADVANTAGES OUTWEIGH THE DISADVANTAGES?

Advantages Outweigh Disadvantages \ Grad Yr	1972	1973	1975	1976	Total
Yes	19 (100)	29 (93)	47 (73)	53 (80)	148 (82)
No	0	2 (7)	17 (27)	13 (20)	32 (18)
Total	19	31	64	66	180

Missing Observations = 12

* Percentages for all tables are given in brackets

IF YOU WERE TO BEGIN YOUR MEDICAL SCHOOL YEARS AGAIN, WHICH OF THE FOLLOWING
TYPES OF PROGRAMS WOULD APPEAL TO YOU?

	Five years out		Two Years Out			
Program Appeal	1972	1973	1975	1976	TOTAL	
Traditional Program Completed in 4 Years	0	0	1 (1)	0	1	(.5)
4-Year Program that allowed me to study topics in the traditional fashion and offered the option of studying topics in small groups.	1 (5)*	1 (3)	7 (11)	6 (8)	15	(8)
Traditional Program Completed in 3 Years	0	1 (3)	2 (3)	1 (1)	4	(2)
3-Year Traditional Program that offered the option of studying topics individually or in small groups	2 (11)	7 (20)	19 (29)	12 (17)	40	(21)
The 3-Year Program at McMaster	16 (84)	23 (66)	31 (48)	46 (64)	116	(61)
Other Type of Program	0	3 (8)	5 (8)	7 (10)	15	(8)
Total	19	35	65	72	191	

Missing Observations = 1

*   Percentages are given in brackets

OVERALL, HOW PREPARED WERE YOU FOR YOUR INTERNSHIP OR FIRST YEAR RESIDENCY
COMPARED WITH OTHER FIRST POSTGRADUATE YEAR TRAINEES YOU ENCOUNTERED?

Grad Yr / Compared to Other Interns	Five Years Out		Two Years Out		Total
	1972	1973	1975	1976	
Much Better Prepared	0	1 (3)*	3 (5)	1 (1)	5 (3)
Better Prepared	5 (26)	7 (20)	11 (17)	17 (23)	40 (21)
About the Same	13 (68)	22 (63)	37 (58)	49 (67)	121 (63)
Less Prepared	1 (5)	5 (14)	11 (17)	6 (8)	23 (12)
Much Less Prepared	0	0	2 (3)	0	2 (1)
Total	19	35	64	73	191

Missing Observations = 1

* Percentages are given in brackets

APPENDIX C

FACULTY OF HEALTH SCIENCES
McMaster University

ANNOTATED BIBLIOGRAPHY

FACULTY OF HEALTH SCIENCES
McMaster University
ANNOTATED BIBLIOGRAPHY

GENERAL

McMaster in the 70's. Published by the Department of Information and
Publications and the Community and Public Relations Office, McMaster
University, Hamilton, Ontario.
A pamphlet commemorating the opening of the on-campus Health Sciences
Centre, describing the relationship between form and function in a
building designed to accommodate both an independent hospital and a
faculty of health sciences.

Mustard, J.F. The Faculty of Health Sciences at McMaster University.
In Health, Higher Education and the Community. Paris, France, OECD
Publications, 1977. p. 199-210.
A description of the internal organization of the Faculty of Health
Sciences, its policies and objectives, its relationships within the
community, and the nature of its programs in education, research
and health services.

Additional References

Campbell, E.J.M. McMaster University and medicine. J. Royal College of
Physicians London 5:332-43, July 1972.
An overview of the School of Medicine and its relationship to
McMaster University.

Evans, J.R. Organizational patterns for new responsibilities. Journal of
Medical Education 45:988-999, 1970.
An early description of the goals of the Faculty of Health Sciences,
and a description of the organizational arrangements to meet the
varied goals of the faculty.

Fraenkel, G.J. McMaster Revisited. British Medical Journal 2:1072-76,
14 Oct. 1978.
A critique by the visiting dean of an Australian medical school of
the McMaster program after ten years of experience.

Hamilton-Wentworth District Health Library Network. Annual Report.
The annual report of the Health Library Network in Hamilton which
includes various tables and descriptive statistics.

Lee, Betty Lou. McMaster builds a fitting home. Canadian Medical
Assoc. J. 107:574-77, 1973.
An article written at the time of the official opening of the
McMaster University Health Sciences Centre, describing the new
facility.

Maastricht and McMaster. *Metamedica* 74(10) 1974. 22p.
A report of the new Faculty of Medicine at Maastricht, Holland,
and the similarities between the educational approaches used at
Maastricht and McMaster; the document was based on a visit by a
large number of foundation faculty members of Maastricht to
McMaster in 1973.

Spaulding, W.B. and Neufeld, V.R. Regionalization of medical education
at McMaster University. *British Medical Journal* 3:95-98, July 1973.
A description and various examples of how education is arranged
on a regional basis; examples include the library and the
contribution of physicians in practice to the education of medical
students.

Zeidler, E.H. *Healing the Hospital: McMaster Health Sciences Centre.*
Toronto, Zeidler, 1974.
A book written from the point of view of the architect who designed
the McMaster University Health Sciences Centre; it attempts to
show the harmony between the functions of the Centre and the
architectural structure of the building.

EDUCATION

Hamilton, John D. The McMaster curriculum: a critique. *British Medical
Journal* 1:1191-96, 1976.
This article describes the history and objectives of the McMaster
M.D. Program and its curriculum, appraises its strengths and
problems, and offers suggestions for its application in other
universities.

Neufeld, V.R. and Barrows, H.S. The McMaster philosophy: an approach
to medical education. *J. Med. Education* 49(11): 1040-1050, Nov. 1974.
This paper outlines the goals of the McMaster M.D. Program and the
central set of ideas which forms the basis for the selection process,
the program components, the evaluation system, and the learning
events and resources.

Sibley, J.C. Postgraduate (residency) training at McMaster: a strategy
for change. *Medical Education* 12(5) Suppl. p. 76-81, 1978.
A presentation of the background of developments in postgraduate
education in the Faculty of Health Sciences, its postgraduate
educational objectives, and the strategies used to implement change.

Additional References

Ali, M.A., Thomas, E.J., Hamilton, J.D. and Brain, M.C. Blood and Guts:
one component of an integrated program in biological sciences as
applied to medicine. *Canadian Medical Assoc. J.* 116:59-61, Jan. 1977.
One year of the undergraduate program is organized along the lines
of "organ system units"; this paper describes one of these units.

Dickinson, C.J., Goldsmith, C.H. and Sackett, D.L. MacMan: a digital
computer model for teaching some basic principles of hemodynamics.
J. of Clinical Computing 2(4):42-50, Jan. 1973.
   A description of one of the computer-based physiologic models -
   the cardiovascular model.

Ferrier, B.M., McAuley, R.G. and Roberts, R.S. Selection of medical
students at McMaster University. J. Roy. Coll. Physicians London
12(4):365-78, July 1978.
   An updated description of the system for selecting medical students
   at McMaster University.

Kergin, D.J., Yoshida, M.A., Spitzer, W.O., Davis, J.E., Buzzell, E.M.
Changing nursing practice through education. The Canadian Nurse
69(4):1-4, April 1973.
   This report of McMaster University's program to prepare family
   practice nurses shows that changes in patterns of practice can be made
   through the educational process.

Leeder, S.R. and Sackett, D.L. The medical undergraduate program at
McMaster University. Learning in Epidemiology and Biostatistics in
an integrated curriculum. Medical J. Australia 2:875-881, Dec. 1976.
   A descriptive example of how a "discipline" such as Clinical
   Epidemiology and Biostatistics is integrated into a problem-based
   curriculum.

Neufeld, V.R. and Spaulding, W.B. Use of learning resources at McMaster
University. British Medical Journal 3:99-101, July 1973.
   A summary of how resources such as audio-visual aids, print materials,
   problem-based learning resources, and other resources are used in
   the education programs at McMaster.

P.E.D. Annual Reports 1977/8 and 1979.
   Summaries of the work of the Program for Educational Development -
   the group responsible for research and development in education.

Pallie, W. and Brain, E. "Modules" in morphology for self-study: a
system for learning in an undergraduate medical program. Medical
Education 12:107-113, 1978.
   A paper describing the imaginative contribution of morphologists
   to the education of medical students.

Robinow, Beatrix H. Audiovisuals and non-print learning resources in
a Health Sciences Library. Journal of Biocommunication 6:14-19,
March 1979.

Simpson, M.A. Medical student evaluation in the absence of examinations.
Medical Education 10(1):22-26, 1976.
   A review of the system used in the undergraduate M.D. Program for
   evaluation of student performance.

Spitzer, W.O., Sackett, D.L., Sibley, J.C., Roberts, R.S., Gent, M., Kergin, D.J., Hackett, B.C., Olynich, A. The Burlington randomized trial of the nurse practitioner. New England Journal of Medicine 290:251-256, January 31, 1974.
> A study of the effectiveness of the nurse practitioner, a registered nurse with special training in primary care, in the complementary role of co-practitioner with primary care physicians in the community of Burlington, Ontario.

Sweeney, G.D. and Mitchell, D.L.M. An introduction to the study of medicine: Phase I of the McMaster M.D. Program. J. Med. Education 50:70-77, January 1975.
> A report on how medical students are introduced to their studies at McMaster.

RESEARCH

Bienenstock, J. Role and Functions of the Committee on Scientific Development. Typescript, June, 1979. Available through the Community and Public Relations Office, McMaster University.
> A description of the committee responsible for the development of research policy and the administration of research in the Faculty of Health Sciences.

Gent, M., Leeder, S.R. and Sackett, D.L. Making research relevant. Med. J. Australia 2:807-12, Dec. 10, 1977.
> A review of the collaborative medical and health care research carried out by the Department of Clinical Epidemiology and Biostatistics at McMaster between 1970 and 1976.

Mustard, J.F. Health research and graduate education. J. Royal College of Physicians London 6:373-79, July 1972.
> A description of the research policies and objectives established by the Faculty of Health Sciences, the mechanisms for administration, coordination and funding, and the development of graduate programs which carry out its research objectives.

Additional References

Bienenstock, J. Host resistance between friends. J. Royal College of Physicians London 6:407-11, July, 1972.
> A description of an interdisciplinary research program in immunology.

Hirsh, J. and Regoeczi, E. Thromboembolism and haemostasis programme. J. Royal College of Physicians London 6:399-406, July 1972.
> Another description of an interdisciplinary research program that has educational and service components as well.

HEALTH SERVICES

Brain, M.C. The Hamilton District Program in Laboratory Medicine: a progress report on integration. Canad. Med. Assoc. J. 114:721-26, April. 17, 1976.

A comprehensive report on how the district-wide program in laboratory medicine is conceived, implemented and evaluated.

Brandstater, M.E. Rehabilitation. J. Royal College of Physicians London 6:415-18, July 1972.

An earlier report on how rehabilitation services and training in rehabilitation medicine are organized in Hamilton.

Robinow, Beatrix H. Hamilton-Wentworth District Health Library Network. Canadian Health Libraries Association Newsletter no.5, Spring 1978 p. 15-17.

A report on the establishment of a cooperative health library network within the McMaster Health Care Region.

student, 74; student mix, data on, 68-69]; problems of medical schools, addressing, 3-5; promotion and recognition of faculty, 6; Residency Program in Family Medicine, 82; student mix, desired, 65, 68-69, [data on, 68-69]; Undergraduate Medicine program, 2

Michigan State University, 50

Miller, George, 49, 61, 62

Montreal Children's Hospital, 76, 77

motivation (see faculty motivation; faculty recruitment, student motivation)

Mustard, Dr. J. Fraser, 19, 31, 62

mutagens, 5

Neufeld, Vic, 61

Newcastle, University of, medical school, 25, 27, 32, 116-17, 118, 125, 129

Northwestern University, 119

nurse practitioners, 117-18

OMERAD (Office for Medical Education Research and Development), 50

Ontario Council of Health, 9, 18, 95

Ontario Department of Health, Health Resources Development Plan of, Regional Service Program, 41, 109, 111

Organization for Economic Cooperation and Development, 11, 18, 101; Council, 16, 18; Expert Committee (1975), 16, 18

primary care, 10, 11

problem-based learning, 5, 51, 52-54, 56, 59, 60, 70, 73, 78,

84, 113, 114; developing curriculum for, 53-54, 62-67; resistance to, 53; (see also self-directed learning)

Program for Educational Development, 39, 85, 90, 91, 107

Prywes, Moshe, 51

public health, 10, 127

Public Health Unit, 4

Querido, Dr. A., 92, 117

Regan, Dr. Peter, 122, 127, 128

Regional Service Program (Ontario), 41, 109, 111

regionalization of health services, 18

research at McMaster School of Medicine, 5, 36-45; affiliated hospitals, role of, 40-41; collaborative programs beyond local community, 42-43; Committee on Scientific Development (C.S.D.), 36-37, 40; community activities, 41-42, [Regional Service Program, 41-42, 109, 111]; interaction with education, graduate programs for, 43-45; other University components, joint efforts with, 40; Program for Educational Development, 39, 85, 90, 91, 107; programs and areas for, 37-39; Rose Levy Rosenstadt Scholar Award, 45

research in health sciences networks, 108-12; factors and biases influencing problem choice, 110-11, [ideology, 110; money, 110; personal charisma, 110-11]; meaning of research, 108-09, 112; organization of the, 111-12; role of a network university, 109; who should do, 111

Rosinsky, 49
Royal College of Physicians and
Surgeons, 79
Royal Commission on the National
Health Services, Report of
(1979), 20

Sackett, Dr. David, 43
St. Joseph's Hospital, 5
Schmidt, Henk G., 47
School of Medicine, McMaster
University (see Medicine,
School of [McMaster Univer-
sity])
self-care, 10, 11
self-directed learning, 5, 50-51,
60, 63-64, 70, 72, 73, 84,
116 (see also problem-based
learning)
self-learning (see self-directed
learning)
Sharpe, Gladys, 1
Shaw, George Bernard, 33
Sibley, Dr. Jack, 101
Spaulding, Dr. William, 62,
68, 82, 86
student motivation, 129-30

Taba, A. H., 55-56
Taylor, Wayne, 43
teacher preparation, 32-33
teaching, relation of, to health
care, 19-20, 21
Terris, Milton, 58
Texas College of Osteopathic
Medicine, 117

Thode, President Harry, 2,
3, 121
Tiddens, Dr. Harmen, 118
Todd Report (1968, Great
Britain), 18
Toronto, University of, 1, 42,
63, 68
Toronto Western Hospital, 1

Updike, John, aphorism on
problems, 93

Virchow, Rudolf, 96

Walsh, Dr. William, 1, 62,
63, 82
Waterloo, University of, 42
Western Ontario, University
of, 42, 63
Westlund, Professor Knut,
106
White, Dr. Kerr L., 23, 114,
122, 127
Wilde, Oscar, aphorism on
learning, 100
Woodward, Dr. Christel, 76
World Bank, 122
World Health Organization
(WHO), 10, 22, 55, 61,
124; Alma-Ata meeting, 11,
22; Fourth Regional Seminar
on Education and Training
for Deans of Medical Schools
in the Western Pacific Region, 30; teacher training
program, 49